Practical
Endocrinology

Practical Endocrinology

NELSON B. WATTS, M.D.
Associate Professor of Medicine (Endocrinology)
Emory University School of Medicine
Atlanta, Georgia

JOSEPH H. KEFFER, M.D.
Medical Director
Nichols Institute Network
San Juan Capistrano, California

Fourth Edition

Lea & Febiger

1989   Philadelphia   London

Lea & Febiger
600 Washington Square
Philadelphia, PA   19106-4198
U.S.A.
(215) 922-1330

The first edition of this book was titled *Modern Solutions to Common Endocrinologic Problems* by Keffer and Watts. It was published in 1975 by Precision Diagnostic Press, Asheville, North Carolina.

First Edition, 1975
Second Edition, 1978
Third Edition, 1982
Fourth Edition, 1989

LIBRARY OF CONGRESS
Library of Congress Cataloging-in-Publication Data

Watts, Nelson B., 1944–
    Practical endocrinology / Nelson B. Watts, Joseph H. Keffer.—
4th ed.
        p.   cm.
    Rev. ed. of: Practical endocrine diagnosis / Nelson B. Watts,
Joseph H. Keffer. 3rd ed. 1982.
    Includes bibliographies and index.
    ISBN 0-8121-1179-6
    1. Endocrinology. 2. Endocrine glands—Diseases. 3. Endocrine
glands—Pathophysiology. 4. Hormones—Analysis. I. Keffer, Joseph H.
II. Watts, Nelson B., 1944–   Practical endocrine diagnosis.
III. Title.
    [DNLM: 1. Endocrine Diseases—diagnosis. 2. Endocrine Diseases—
therapy. WK 100 W352p]
RC649.W37   1989
616.4'0756—dc19
DNLM/DLC   88-8206
for Library of Congress   CIP

Printed in the United States of America

Print number: 5   4   3   2   1

PREFACE

This book began in 1974 with the first of an ongoing series of workshops for the American Society of Clinical Pathologists entitled *Modern Solutions to Common Endocrinologic Problems.* The impetus came from everyday clinical situations. We found that most of the diagnostic questions we encountered in practice could be solved by open communication between the clinician (Watts) and the laboratorian (Keffer), applying protocols gleaned from the literature with assays that could be done in a general clinical laboratory. Often, it was hard to get all the specific details essential for performance and interpretation of the tests.

The first edition of this book emphasized specific diagnostic protocols and assay methodology. At the time, most of the protocols we presented seemed "new," even though some had been published more than 10 years before! The assay methods often seemed complex and intimidating, yet most of the reagents were commercially available and the equipment was affordable. Through the second and third editions, the emphasis shifted away from assay methodology (as these techniques became accepted in clinical laboratories) and focused more on diagnostic protocols. Now, most of these protocols have achieved general acceptance and availability. In addition to updating the material from the previous work, this fourth edition includes added material on pathophysiology and, for the first time, information on the treatment of endocrine disorders. The new title, *Practical Endocrinology,* indicates the expanded focus.

As with previous editions, this manual should add to the ease and accuracy with which endocrine diagnoses are made, providing the criteria for selection of tests and protocols for testing. The new material should add to the understanding of disease processes and help in deciding appropriate treatment. We have not attempted to be comprehensive in the areas we have covered, choosing to focus on practical approaches to common problems. In doing so, we have reviewed the more comprehensive sources and selectively endorsed elements that are most productive. Reading from cover to cover should be informative but not necessary. We hope that the reader can extract the material pertinent to his or her patient, or to the problem at hand, with a minimum of distraction.

Atlanta, GA   Nelson B. Watts
San Juan Capistrano, CA   Joseph H. Keffer

CONTENTS

1

Basic Concepts

Endocrinology is the study of hormones, substances produced in one organ and transported through the blood stream to distant target tissues. While diabetes mellitus and thyroid diseases make up the majority of problems seen in clinical endocrinology, there are a host of additional areas that present challenges. This subspecialty of internal medicine and pediatrics allows one to apply knowledge from the basic science disciplines (anatomy, physiology, biochemistry, etc.,) to the diagnosis and treatment of patients. Most hormones can be measured with a high degree of accuracy and relative ease, providing confirmation of clinical assessment, and, in many instances, clarifying suspicions that could not be answered any other way. Most patients with endocrine disorders can be restored to normal or near normal function, with the end result being highly rewarding for patient and physician alike.

There are three areas of importance when evaluating patients known or suspected to have an endocrine disorder: (1) basic fund of knowledge regarding normal physiology, pathophysiology, and the natural history of specific endocrine diseases; (2) command of basic clinical skills (history and physical examination), with the ability to focus appropriately on the diagnostic possibilities; and (3) understanding the strengths and limitations of studies used to investigate endocrine disorders, particularly hormone measurements.

The purpose of this chapter is to provide a review and overview of concepts that are important for understanding the clinical manifestations of endocrine diseases, interpreting the results of diagnostic tests, and planning appropriate therapy. Some previous exposure to this information is assumed; we will not attempt to be comprehensive or detailed in the areas covered. For more extensive or basic information, the reader should consult one of the several excellent textbooks that are available.

Besser GM, Cudworth AG: Clincal Endocrinology: An Illustrated Text. Philadelphia, JB Lippincott, 1987.

Felig P, Baxter JD, Broadus AE et al. (eds): Endocrinology and Metabolism, 2nd ed. New York, McGraw-Hill, 1987.

Wilson JD, Foster DW: Williams' Textbook of Endocrinology, 7th ed. Philadelphia, WB Saunders, 1985.

PHYSIOLOGY

Hormones are involved at different levels (cell, organ, whole organism) and in a variety of processes (growth and differentiation; development, maturation, and reproduction; energy production, utilization, and storage; and control of fluid and electrolyte balance). Disorders of endocrine glands include hormone deficiency and excess states, as well as neoplastic conditions that may or may not affect glandular function.

Regulation of endocrine function includes the following steps: (1) synthesis, (2) storage, (3) secretion, (4) transport, (5) cellular action, and (6) degradation. These steps are coordinated by "signaling" in the form of other hormones (called tropic hormones), the hormone product itself, or nonhormonal factors (Fig. 1–1).

FEEDBACK AND SIGNALING

A particularly important concept in the regulation of endocrine systems is negative feedback (feedback inhibition), where the rising concentration of hormone A inhibits the release of hormone B, the hormone that signals the release of hormone A. Some endocrine systems are "closed loop" feedback, where the output affects the response of the system to input (e.g., thyroid hormone inhibits release of thyroid stimulating hormone from the pituitary gland). "Open loop" feedback systems are present, especially at the cellular level of hormone action, where the input affects the output, but the converse is not true. Many endocrine systems involve multiple steps that are subject to modification by outside influences.

In addition to the effect that one hormone may have on the release or action of another, biologic rhythms and other nonhormonal stimuli may also have effects. Hormone secretion may be episodic or pulsatile, varying over a few minues, a day (circadian, e.g., ACTH and cortisol) or longer (infradian, e.g., the menstrual cycle). Physiologic variables that determine the appropriateness of a specific hormone level are just as important for interpretation of laboratory test results as the precision and accuracy of the assay itself.

2

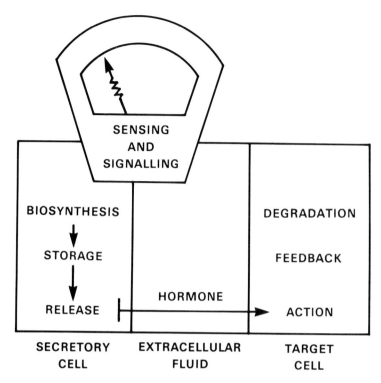

Fig. 1–1. The components of an endocrine system. (Used by permission from Roth J, Grunfeld C: Endocrine systems: Mechanisms of disease, target cells, and receptors. *in* Williams RH (ed): Textbook Of Endocrinology, 6th ed. Philadelphia, WB Saunders, 1981.)

SECRETION, TRANSPORT, AND DEGRADATION

"Prohormone" is the term used to describe a substance of low biologic activity which is converted to a more active configuration. This conversion may take place prior to release of the hormone from the cell of origin (e.g., proinsulin to insulin), in the circulation (e.g., angiotensin I to angiotensin II), or at the level of cellular activity (e.g., testosterone to dihydrotestosterone). If a precursor to a prohormone is identified, it is usually called a "pre-prohormone." This may lead to confusion in terminology as well as confusion in interpretation of assay results.

With regard to protein or polypeptide hormones, fragments of the same hormone of varying size and differing biologic activity may be circulating simultaneously due to cleavage of the intact hormone (e.g., parathyroid hormone, with active intact and N-terminal fragments and inactive C-terminal fragments all found in the circulation). Bioactivity may be influenced by ap-

3

parently minor changes in configuration, such as the sites of glycosylation of thyroid stimulating hormone. When bioactivity and immunoassayable activity of a particular hormone are different, there may be difficulties in the clinical interpretation of laboratory results.

Thyroid hormones and most steroid hormones circulate in blood reversibly bound to high-affinity carrier proteins, as well as loosely bound to albumin. Generally, the bound hormone fraction is biologically inactive, with the free (unbound) fraction being the pool with biologic activity. Changes in the level of binding proteins will affect the total hormone concentration without altering the free (active) fraction.

HORMONE TYPES

There are three main classes of hormones in man: steroid, polypeptide, and amine.

The steroid ring is the basic framework for steroid hormones; specific biologic activity of each hormone is conferred by differences in side chains. The half-lives of steroid hormones are typically 60 to 120 minutes, compared to 10 to 30 minutes for peptide hormones and less than 5 minutes for catecholamines. The steroid hormones include adrenal glucocorticoids, mineralocorticoids, gonadal hormones, and vitamin D metabolites.

Protein (or polypeptide) hormones are made up of amino acids linked together, ranging in size from three to hundreds of amino acids. Often, a small portion on the sequence provides full biologic activity; the inactive part of the molecule may serve to protect the hormone from degradation or to enhance binding to cellular receptors. Hypothalamic hormones, pituitary hormones, parathyroid hormone, and insulin are examples of protein hormones.

The amine hormones include dopamine, norepinephrine, epinephrine, and thyroid hormones.

CELLULAR MECHANISMS OF HORMONE ACTION

Minute quantities of hormone have selective and dramatic influences. In target tissues, the "one in a million" hormone molecule reaches its site of action by virtue of specific receptors on the plasma membrane or in the nucleus of the target cell. Hormone localization in target tissue is a reversible reaction. Receptors have high affinity for their hormone; that is, a great tendency for binding and a minimal tendency to release the

4

hormone. In contrast, serum binding proteins (e.g., thyroxine binding globulin) have lesser affinity than the cellular receptors, so they will readily release their cargo at the appropriate target sites. In addition to high affinity, hormone receptors are highly specific, generally binding with only one hormone in the physiologic range of hormone concentrations. If a hormone that is chemically similar is present in high concentration, "receptor spillover" may occur (e.g., chorionic gonadotropin in high amounts will bind with and activate the receptors for thyroid stimulating hormone).

Adenyl Cyclase

Most polypeptide hormones affect cellular metabolism through the adenyl cyclase system (Fig. 1–2). Circulating hormone binds rapidly and reversibly to a hormone-specific receptor on the surface of the cell membrane. Binding of the hormone to its receptor results in activation of adenyl cyclase, an enzyme that converts adenosine triphosphate (ATP) to 3′,5′-adenosine monophosphate (cyclic AMP). Cyclic AMP is rapidly inactivated; before its degradation, cyclic AMP activates an en-

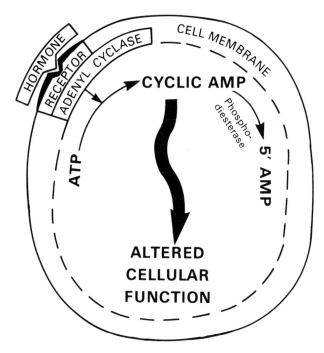

Fig. 1–2. Hormone action through the adenyl cyclase system.

5

zyme kinase system which modifies cellular function. The scheme of the specific hormone as "first messenger" and cyclic AMP as a "second messenger" as outlined above may be similar for hormones such as insulin and growth hormone that do not work through adenyl cyclase but may work through other "second messengers," as yet unidentified.

Steroid Hormone Action

A different concept has been advanced to explain the mechanism of steroid hormone action in cells (Fig. 1–3). Entering the cytoplasm readily, steroid hormones move into the nucleus and bind with their receptors; the hormone-receptor complex

STEROID HORMONE RESPONSIVE CELL

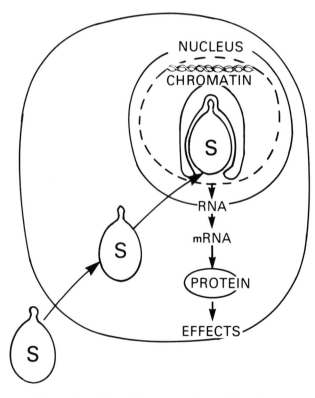

Fig. 1–3. Mechanism of steroid hormone action. (Abbreviations: s = steroid hormone, mRNA = messenger RNA.)

activates nuclear chromatin and induces the formation of messenger RNA, which enters the cytoplasm and increases the synthesis of specific cellular proteins.

Thyroid Hormone Action

Thyroid hormones, like steroid hormones, pass easily through cell membranes. They may be reversibly bound to sites in the cytoplasm, but hormone action begins when the hormone (triiodothyronine) binds to receptors in nuclear chromatin. Triiodothyronine enters the cells by diffusion as well as being derived locally from conversion of thyroxine. The thyroid hormone-receptor combination leads to production of messenger RNA, which in turn affects synthesis of cellular proteins (Fig. 1–4).

Clinical Significance of Hormone Receptors

Changes in hormone receptors may be the cause of disease or the result of disease. A primary deficiency in cell receptors

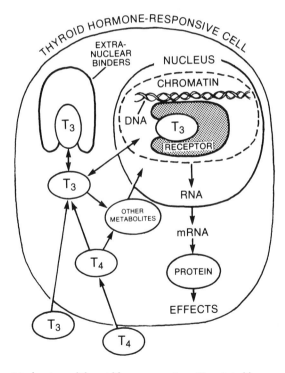

Fig. 1–4. Mechanism of thyroid hormone action. (Reprinted by permission of the New England Journal of Medicine. Baxter JD, Funder JW: Hormone receptors. 1979; *301*:1149.)

accounts for testicular feminization, pseudohypoparathyroidism, and other uncommon conditions. A reduction in insulin receptor number plays a part in the insulin resistance that characterizes patients with obesity and noninsulin-dependent diabetes mellitus. Antibodies to receptors may cause disease (e.g., myasthenia gravis, Graves' hyperthyroidism). Receptor content of tissues may determine their response to drugs (e.g., estrogen and progesterone receptors in breast cancer). One hormone may have multiple sites of origin and multiple actions (e.g., somatostatin, produced in the central nervous system, hypothalamus, and throughout the GI tract, with pronounced effects on the release of other hormones and on gastrointestinal function); conversely, one function may be controlled by multiple hormones (e.g., glucose homeostasis is regulated by insulin and "counterregulatory" hormones including glucagon, epinephrine, cortisol, and growth hormone; control of ovulation by LH, FSH, estrogen, and progesterone).

ENDOCRINE FOCUS ON HISTORY AND PHYSICAL EXAMINATION

Patients are sometimes referred with their diagnosis already suspected or established, or with such a classic and obvious presentation that their diagnosis is apparent. More often, however, patients seek medical attention because of their awareness that something is wrong and rely on the physician to sort out the signs and symptoms. There is no substitute for a complete history and physical examination for beginning the evaluation process. Specific issues that should be sought on review of systems which would suggest endocrine disease include:

1. Change in body weight or configuration; if so, over what time period, and with any change in appetite or activity?
2. Change in skin or hair?
3. Change in reproductive function (amenorrhea, infertility, galactorrhea in women; impotence, infertility in men)?
4. Heat or cold intolerance (thyroid dysfunction)?
5. Palpitations, tachycardia, hypertension (hyperthyroidism, pheochromocytoma)?
6. Nervousness, tremor (hyperthyroidism, pheochromocytoma)?
7. Easy fatigue, muscle weakness, muscle cramps (hyper- or hypothyroidism, Cushing's syndrome, hypercalcemia)?
8. Anxiety, depression, clouded mentation?

Specific aspects of the physical examination that require experience and practice include examination of the thyroid and testing of visual fields. These areas will be discussed again and expanded on in the relevant chapters.

HORMONE ASSAYS AND OTHER ANCILLARY TESTS

Endocrine testing only rarely involves measurement of a single substance. Biologic influences and variations in laboratory sensitivity and precision make it unwise to rely on a single random measurement. Fortunately, it is possible to take advantage of principles of physiology and pathophysiology to develop powerful strategies for testing. At least three general principles are used:

1. Dynamic testing (stimulation and suppression). This is a classic principle of endocrinology; knowing factors that influence hormone secretion, it is possible to manipulate the system and evaluate the response. Does cortisol fall appropriately when sufficient glucocorticoid is provided to suppress ACTH? Does thyroid stimulating hormone (TSH) rise normally after intravenous thyrotropin releasing hormone (TRH)? By manipulating the system in a standard fashion, "normal" and "abnormal" can be defined.

2. "Hormone pairs" (measurement of two parts of a feedback system). With negative feedback, if hormone B falls, hormone A should go up; this is true even if hormone B has not dropped below the lower limit of the "normal" range. This strategy is useful for evaluating the significance of a "borderline" low value (e.g., if T_4 is 5.5 μg/dL, with a reference range of 5.0 to 10.0 μg/dL, an elevated TSH indicates hypothyroidism; a normal TSH in the absence of pituitary or hypothalamic disease indicates euthyroidism). This approach is also useful in deciding if endocrine hypofunction is primary (target gland) or secondary (pituitary or hypothalamus) (e.g., if cortisol is low, high ACTH indicates primary adrenal gland failure, low ACTH suggests pituitary or hypothalamic problems).

3. Multivariate (or bivariate) analysis. This approach presents one value in the perspective of at least one other variable. This has come to be accepted as standard for measurements such as parathyroid hormone, which can only be interpreted if serum calcium (ideally, ionized calcium) and renal function are known, or with insulin levels, which cannot be evaluated without knowing simultaneous glucose levels.

An ideal assay would be accurate (measuring what is stated,

9

close to the absolute value) and precise (reproducible within a narrow range). Deviation from this ideal may limit or exclude the use of a particular assay for one disease, yet be of little significance in another. For example, until recently, TSH measurement was not sensitive enough to be useful for the diagnosis of hyperthyroidism, but TSH is excellent for the diagnosis of hypothyroidism. Other desirable qualities in an assay are low cost, simplicity (the ability to be performed by persons with limited skills), and rapid turn-around.

Most hormone measurements today involve the principle of *immunoassay*. The explosion in knowledge of endocrine physiology could never have proceeded so rapidly without this technique. These assays rely on the use of antibodies as reagents; the specific characteristics of the antibody will determine if significant cross-reactivity will occur. For some time, the generation of antibodies for assays was its own special art; however, with the availability of monoclonal antibodies, standard (though not necesarily better) antibodies in large supply should simplify problems with interlaboratory comparison of results. Initially, immunoassays were performed using radioactive isotopes as indicators (specifically called radioimmunoassay, or RIA). Now, enzyme reactions have begun to replace radioisotopes, with fluorometry or other techniques used to measure the end point. Nonisotopic immunoassays can be expected to replace the bulk of the applications involving the radioisotope because of the longer shelf life, inherent economic advantages, and the avoidance of regulatory controls (particularly the expense of radioisotope disposal).

Bioassays evaluate an effect of a hormone in one of its target tissues. Bioassays are rarely used today in clinical practice for a variety of reasons. Problems of interpreting bioassays include differing responses depending on the target tissue and end point selected and the existence of circulating substances that inhibit action of the hormone.

2

Anterior Pituitary and Hypothalamus

INTRODUCTION, BACKGROUND, NORMAL PHYSIOLOGY

The pituitary gland is located at the base of the brain just below the optic chiasm and just above the sphenoid sinus. It is divided into two lobes. The anterior lobe is supplied with blood by a venous portal system that contains hormonal regulating substances from the hypothalamus. The posterior lobe is innervated by nerve fibers that originate in the hypothalamus. The importance of the anterior pituitary gland in the regulation of endocrine function has long been recognized; for many years, the pituitary gland was considered the "conductor of the endocrine orchestra." It is now clear that the pituitary gland is subservient to influences from the hypothalamus which stimulate or inhibit the release of anterior pituitary hormones.

HORMONES OF THE ANTERIOR PITUITARY GLAND

The anterior pituitary gland contains five types of cells. Four cell types each produce a different hormone—growth hormone (GH), prolactin (PRL), thyroid stimulating hormone (TSH), and adrenocorticortropic hormone (ACTH), while a fifth cell type produces two related hormones—the gonadotropins, luteinizing hormone (LH) and follicle-stimulating hormone (FSH). Table 2–1 summarizes these hormones, their respective hypothalamic factors, and their target organs. PRL and GH have diffuse actions throughout the body. In contrast, the other hormones of the anterior pituitary act primarily on distant endocrine organs and are regulated in part by the products of their target glands. These target glands are the thyroid gland, the adrenal glands, and the gonads.

Hormone Structure

The hormones of the anterior pituitary gland can be divided into two groups based on their structure. GH, PRL, and ACTH

11

Table 2–1. Anterior Pituitary Hormones

Hormone	Structure	Hypothalamic Factor	Target Tissue
GH	protein	GHRH (s),* SRIF (i)†	bone, soft tissue
PRL	protein	dopamine (i)	breast
ACTH	protein	CRH (s)	adrenal cortex
LH	glycoprotein	GnRH (s)	gonads (steroid-producing cells)
FSH	glycoprotein	GnRH (s)	gonads (gamete-producing cells)
TSH	glycoprotein	TRH (s)	thyroid gland

*(s) = stimulatory
†(i) = inhibitory
Abbreviations: GH, growth hormone; GHRH, growth hormone releasing hormone; SRIF, somatostatin; PRL, prolactin; ACTH, adrenocorticotropic hormone; CRH, corticotropin releasing hormone; LH, luteinizing hormone; GnRH, gonadotropin releasing hormone; FSH, follicle stimulating hormone; TSH, thyroid stimulating hormone; TRH, thyrotropin releasing hormone.
(Used with permission from Watts NB: Pituitary dysfunction: Clinical effects and hormone assays. Laboratory Management 1986; *24*:53–60)

are *protein* hormones (191, 199, and 39 amino acids in size, respectively). GH is similar in structure to PRL and almost identical to the placental hormone chorionic somatomammotropin. PRL is similar to another placental hormone, human placental lactogen. LH, FSH, and TSH are made up of identical alpha subunits, and unique beta subunits that confer specific biologic activity to these hormones. Both subunits contain carbohydrate in addition to their basic protein structure, thus the name *glycoprotein* hormones. Another placental hormone, *chorionic gonadotropin* (hCG), is similar in structure to LH.

Control of Secretion

The secretion of each of these hormones is controlled through complex mechanisms that include regulatory hormones from the hypothalamus (Table 2–1). PRL release is inhibited by a hypothalamic factor which appears to be dopamine. The other anterior pituitary hormones (TSH, ACTH, LH, FSH, and GH) are regulated primarily by stimulatory factors from the hypothalamus. GH appears to be unique in also having an inhibitory hypothalamic hormone (somatostatin).

GH and PRL will be discussed in more detail in this chapter.

TSH, ACTH, and the gonadotropins will be mentioned here but treated in detail in other chapters.

Thyroid stimulating hormone (TSH) acts on the thyroid gland to increase the synthesis and release of thyroid hormones, thyroxine (T_4) and triiodothyronine (T_3), as well as to promote growth of thyroid cells. Thyroid hormones exert an inhibitory effect on the pituitary; TSH release is suppressed by a slight increase in thyroid hormones and rises exponentially as thyroid hormone levels decrease. TSH secretion is pulsatile within a narrow range (0.5 to 4.0 mU/L) and shows a diurnal variation (slightly higher at night).

Adrenocorticotropic hormone (ACTH) is a protein of 39 amino acids derived from a large precursor molecule, pro-opiomelanocortin (POMC), which is also the precursor for lipotropin, endorphins, and enkephalins. The ACTH molecule includes the 13 amino acid sequence of melanocyte-stimulating hormone (MSH) and in high concentrations may cause darkening of the skin, as seen in some patients with primary adrenal insufficiency (Addison's disease). ACTH stimulates the adrenal glands to synthesize and release steroid hormones, primarily cortisol. There is negative feedback between the adrenal glands and the pituitary; an increase in cortisol leads to diminished ACTH secretion and a fall in cortisol causes increased ACTH release. Stress is a potent stimulus for ACTH release and will override feedback inhibition. ACTH exhibits a diurnal rhythm, with high values (up to 80 pg/mL) in the early morning hours and low values (<10 pg/mL) in the later afternoon and evening. Cortisol secretion parallels this diurnal rhythm of ACTH.

Luteinizing hormone (LH) and follicle stimulating hormone (FSH). The relationship between the gonadotropins and the gonads is quite complex. A simple generalization is that LH stimulates sex steroid synthesis and is inhibited by rising levels of gonadal steroids. FSH stimulates gametogenesis; feedback on FSH is exerted by sex steroids and possibly by other factors produced by the gonads. In adults, both LH and FSH are released in pulses every 1 to 2 hours. The concentrations of both of these hormones in adults is 5 to 10 mU/L, with high values in women at the middle of the menstrual cycle and after the menopause, and low values in children.

Tindall GT, Barrow DL: Disorders of the Pituitary. St. Louis, CV Mosby, 1986.
Chattoraj SC, Watts NB: Anterior pituitary hormones, pp. 1017–1032, *in* Tietz NW (ed): Textbook of Clinical Chemistry. Philadelphia, WB Saunders, 1986.

Wilson JD, Foster DW (eds): Williams' Textbook of Endocrinology, (7th Ed). Philadelphia, WB Saunders, 1985.

PITUITARY TUMORS

The most common tumors in the area of the pituitary are those that arise from cells of the anterior pituitary, although a wide variety of other tumors are also found (craniopharyngioma, meningioma, sarcoma, etc). Only rarely are pituitary tumors malignant (though some are locally invasive), but considerable morbidity may result from expansion of a benign sellar mass. For anterior pituitary tumors, a variety of classifications have been used. One in general use is based on size: arbitrarily tumors less than 1 cm in diameter are microadenomas, and tumors 1 cm or larger are macroadenomas. Other classifications are based on presumed function of the cell of origin. Standard histology with hematoxylin and eosin shows three cell types: (1) acidophils or eosinophilic cells, thought to contain either GH or PRL; (2) basophils, containing either ACTH, TSH, LH, or FSH; and (3) chromophobes, for years thought to be hormonally inactive. A more recently accepted classification is based on immunohistochemistry (staining tissue sections with antibodies to specific hormones). Many of the chromophobe tumors are found to contain intact hormones or alpha subunits; these "active" chromophobes cannot be distinguished from "null-cell" tumors any other way. Table 2–2 shows the prevalence of the different types of anterior pituitary tumors based on immunohistochemistry. It should be noted that not all tumors that contain hormones will secrete them (e.g., many "chromophobe" tumors contain LH or FSH but blood levels are not always high), and not all tumors that secrete hormones are accompanied by a syndrome of hormone excess (e.g., some pro-

Table 2–2. Types and Prevalence of Anterior Pituitary Tumors

Prevalence (% of Total)	Cell Type (Immunohistochemistry)
30	Prolactin
20	Growth hormone
10	Mixed, PRL and GH
20	None ("Null Cell")
15	ACTH
3	LH, FSH, or both
2	TSH

lactin-secreting tumors are "silent"). While immunohistochemistry and electron microscopy add a special dimension to the evaluation of pituitary tumors, the results do not usually alter clinical management.

The presence of a secretory pituitary tumor is usually suspected because of the manifestations of pituitary hormone excess. These excess states include ACTH (Cushing's syndrome), PRL (amenorrhea and galactorrhea), GH (acromegaly), and rarely, excessive production of TSH or gonadotropins. Frequently these tumors are small when first discovered (microadenomas, <1 cm diameter). The clinical syndromes associated with these functioning pituitary tumors and specific strategies for diagnosis will be discussed further for each specific hormone. In general, a single hormone measurement is unlikely to be conclusive in establishing an excess state because normal fluctuations can cause transient high levels. Agents can be given that would normally suppress these hormones or their target glands; a persistent elevation despite conditions of suppression indicates an abnormality. The agents most commonly used to test pituitary reserve and suppressibility are shown in Table 2–3.

Many anterior pituitary tumors do not produce hormones or do not show clinical evidence of hormone excess. The manifestations of these nonsecreting tumors are usually related to the effects of the expanding mass lesion; for this reason, nonsecretory pituitary adenomas are usually larger than functioning pituitary tumors when they are first discovered. Other mass lesions in the area of the pituitary or hypothalamus, such as craniopharyngiomas, meningiomas, metastatic malignancy, or

Table 2–3. Stimulation and Suppression Tests

Hormone	Suppression	Stimulation
PRL	L-dopa,* bromocriptine*	TRH,* domperidone,* phenothiazines*
LH, FSH	Estrogens, testosterone	GnRH,* clomiphene*
TSH	T_4, T_3	TRH
ACTH	Dexamethasone	Insulin-hypoglycemia, metyrapone, CRH
GH	Oral glucose	Insulin-hypoglycemia, arginine, L-dopa, glucagon, GHRH

*limited clinical usefulness
(Used with permission from Watts NB: Pituitary dysfunction: Clinical effects and hormone assays. Lab Manag 1986; *24*:53–60)

aneurysms, may have a clinical presentation similar to nonsecretory pituitary tumors. The symptoms and signs include headache, visual changes (diplopia, visual field constriction), cranial nerve palsies (III, IV, and VI), and manifestations of hypopituitarism (hypoadrenalism, hypothyroidism, reproductive dysfunction, and/or diabetes insipidus).

Diagnosis of a nonsecretory pituitary tumor rests on the presenting signs and symptoms (usually visual changes, sometimes hypopituitarism) and neuroradiologic techniques. High-resolution computed tomography (CT) can show most lesions >5 mm in diameter, and most nonsecretory tumors are >10 mm. Magnetic resonance imaging (MRI) may permit visualization of even smaller tumors or better anatomic delineation of larger ones. Appropriate tests of endocrine function are outlined in the next section. Complete history and physical examination are important. The classic ocular finding is bitemporal hemianopsia due to upward extension of a tumor. Visual fields should be checked using direct confrontation (the patient covers each eye, one at a time, and is asked to count fingers or spot a small moving object such as a cotton swab in the peripheral fields). In addition, color discrimination should be checked. To do this, the patient covers each eye, one at a time, and looks at two brightly colored items (such as the red tops of eyedrop bottles) simultaneously, one in the nasal field and one in the temporal field, and compares the color intensity in the two fields. If a large tumor is found, formal visual field mapping should be done by an ophthalmologist. Pallor of the optic disc should be looked for.

Treatment of nonsecretory (chromophobe) adenomas depends on the extent of the tumor. Surgery is usually indicated; even when complete resection of the tumor is not possible due to upward extension or to tumor spread laterally into the cavernous sinuses, debulking of the tumor may help restore some vision and endocrine function, as well as provide a smaller field for external irradiation. *Transsphenoidal surgery* was reintroduced in the 1960s and is the preferred approach for almost all pituitary tumors and tumors in the region of the sella. The surgical anatomy of the transsphenoidal approach is shown in Figure 2–1. In the hands of an experienced surgeon, this approach has almost no mortality and minimal morbidity (less than 10% hypopituitarism, CSF leak, meningitis, or optic nerve damage). Most patients are home from the hospital in 6 to 8 days after transsphenoidal surgery and back to full activity in 3 to 4 weeks. For large tumors, this approach may need to be

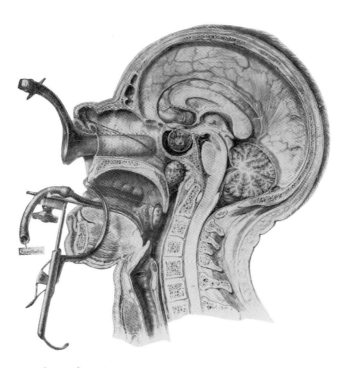

Fig. 2–1. Surgical anatomy of the pituitary: transsphenoidal approach. (Reproduced by permission from Tindall GT, Barrow DL: Disorders of the Pituitary. St. Louis, 1986, The C.V. Mosby Co.)

followed by a subfrontal or subtemporal craniotomy for more complete tumor removal. External irradiation (5000 to 5500 rads) usually halts or slows tumor growth; however, radiation requires a relatively long time before the beneficial effects are seen (often 2 to 4 years), and there are serious delayed risks of radiation including hypopituitarism, cataracts, optic nerve damage, and CNS tumors. Conventional radiation should be reserved for treatment of patients with surgically incurable or recurrent tumors or when surgery cannot be performed because of poor health. Implantation of radioactive seeds may be done if a sufficient dose of external irradiation cannot be delivered safely. Medical therapy is generally ineffective for controlling the growth of nonsecretory tumors (but replacement therapy should be given if hormone deficiencies are present).

Arafah BM: Reversible hypopituitarism in patients with large nonfunctioning pituitary adenomas. J Clin Endocrinol Metab 1986; 62:1173–1179.

Kohler PO: Treatment of pituitary adenomas. N Engl J Med 1987; *317*:45–46.

Melmed S (moderator): Pituitary tumors secreting growth hormone and prolactin. Ann Intern Med 1986; *105*:238–253.

Tindall GT, Hoffman JC: Evaluation of the abnormal sella turcica. Arch Intern Med 1980; *140*:1078–1083.

Zervas NT, Martin JB: Management of hormone-secreting pituitary adenomas. N Engl J Med 1980; *302*:210–214.

TESTING ANTERIOR PITUITARY RESERVE

Abnormalities of pituitary hormones may be single or multiple, deficiency or excess. There is no single test of "pituitary function"; one must test specifically for the hormone(s) of interest. Often (but not invariably), pituitary hormones are lost in reverse order of teleologic importance: growth hormone first, gonadotropins second, thyrotropin third, and ACTH last. Patients with pituitary adenomas are the largest group for whom testing of pituitary function is indicated. Large tumors may cause compression and destruction of normal pituitary tissue, resulting in deficiencies of one, several, or all of the anterior pituitary hormones. Infiltrative or infectious disorders such as sarcoidosis may also compromise pituitary function. Another cause, less common now than in the past, is postpartum pituitary necrosis (Sheehan's syndrome). In addition to testing for hormone reserve in patients with pituitary tumors and suspected hypopituitarism, other situations where anterior pituitary reserve shoud be evaluated include children with short stature (to evaluate the possibility of GH deficiency), and testing for ACTH reserve in patients who have been treated with glucocorticoids.

Initially, anterior pituitary hormones were measured by bioassay. Currently, all of these hormones can be readily measured by immunoassay, some by radioimmunoassay (RIA) and others more easily and precisely by nonisotopic techniques. Because of the normal fluctuations of most of these hormones and the limited sensitivity of most generally available immunoassays in the lower ranges, it had not been possible to distinguish abnormally low levels from the lower range of normal with a high degree of confidence. Commonly, pharmacologic or physiologic stimuli for the release of these hormones have been employed for diagnostic use of suspected hormone deficiency states (Table 2–3). Since the anterior pituitary hormones generally function independently of one another, a test that evaluates one hormone cannot be used to infer the state of others.

Clinically significant anterior pituitary hormone deficiencies that should be tested for include TSH, ACTH, and gonadotropins in children and adults, as well as GH in children. Table 2–3 shows the recommended screening tests for each hormone. Satisfactory information can be obtained with basal measurements of prolactin, gonadotropins, sex hormones (testosterone in males, estradiol in females), thyroxine (T_4), and TSH, along with a rapid ACTH test (cosyntropin test) (protocol, p. 207). Reassessment of endocrine function after pituitary surgery is desirable, although it may be necessary to wait several weeks after surgery for valid results due to transient changes induced by surgery. After pituitary surgery, we find the AM serum cortisol drawn prior to hospital discharge to be a good predictor of pituitary ACTH reserve, and defer retesting thyroid and gonadal axes until the patient returns a month later for followup. An algorithm for testing ACTH reserve after pituitary surgery is shown in Figure 2–2. Specific protocols for testing and criteria for interpretation of other pituitary hormone tests are available (Watts NB, Clark RV. Endocrinological testing in patients with pituitary tumors. Contemporary Neurosurgery 1985; 7:1–6) and should be followed. More details on testing specific hormone reserve can be found in this chapter under each hormone.

Normal target gland function indicates that there is no gross abnormality of pituitary function. For practical purposes, evidence of normal reproductive, thyroid, and/or adrenal gland function may obviate the need for further testing.

By looking for the expected physiologic change in pituitary hormones when there is altered target gland status, pituitary hormone measurements can be quite useful for evaluating target gland dysfunction. Pituitary disorders are uncommon, but failure of target glands (particularly the thyroid, but also the gonads and adrenals) is much more frequent. When function of the target gland is low and the corresponding pituitary hormone is elevated, the problem lies in the target gland. If the pituitary hormone level is "normal" or low in the face of target gland deficiency, the problem is central (pituitary or hypothalamus). Combined assessment of target gland status, basal measurement of pituitary hormones, and responses of pituitary hormones to administration of hypothalamic releasing factors (such as TRH, CRH, GnRH, GHRH), or other stimulatory tests provides a powerful method to assess endocrine function.

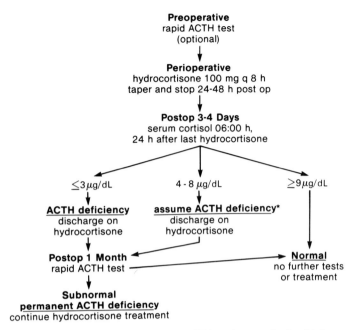

Abbreviations: ITT = insulin tolerance test, ACTH = adrenocorticotrophic hormone

*Consider insulin tolerance test if morning serum cortisol is in this range.

Fig. 2–2. Assessment of adrenal reserve after pituitary surgery. (Used with permission from Watts NB, Tindall GT: Rapid assessment of corticotropin reserve after pituitary surgery. JAMA 1988; *259*:708–711; copyright 1988, the American Medical Assocation.)

Replacement therapy for TSH deficiency is thyroid hormone (L-thyroxine, average dose 0.75 μg/pound of body weight/day); and for ACTH deficiency, hydrocortisone (typically 20 mg each morning, 10 mg each afternoon, increased for stress). For further details on thyroid and adrenal replacement, please read those chapters. Replacement for gonadotropin deficiency depends on the clinical situation; sex hormone replacement (cyclic estrogen and progesterone in females, testosterone in males) is usually chosen, unless fertility is the goal, in which case gonadotropins (chorionic gonadotropin for LH, menopausal gonadotropins for FSH) are given to induce ovulation or spermatogenesis. Growth hormone is given to GH deficient children with short stature.

Daughaday WH: The anterior pituitary, pp 568–613, *in* Wilson JD, Foster DW (eds): Williams' Textbook of Endocrinology, 7th Ed. Philadelphia, WB Saunders, 1985.
Sheldon WR, DeBold CR, Evans WS, et al.: Rapid sequential intrave-

nous administration of four hypothalamic releasing hormones as a combined anterior pituitary function test in normal subjects. J Clin Endocrinol Metab 1985; 60:623–630.

Watts NB, Clark RV: Endocrinological testing in patients with pituitary tumors. Contemporary Neurosurgery 1985; 7:1–6.

Watts NB, Tindall GT: Rapid assessment of ACTH reserve after pituitary surgery. JAMA 1988; 259:708–711.

PROLACTIN

The main role of prolactin in normal physiology is to enhance the production of milk in breast tissue that has already been "primed" by estrogen and progesterone. In vitro, prolactin has effects on salt and water metabolism as well as some androgenic properties, but these actions are usually not of clinical significance.

Background, Pathophysiology

PRL deficiency is not usually clinically important (there are case reports of failure of lactation due to PRL deficiency), and is uncommon as an isolated finding. Agents that normally increase the release of PRL (TRH, insulin, and phenothiazines) can be used to test PRL reserve, but these tests are rarely needed in clinical practice.

PRL excess is common, and may be due to a variety of causes including pituitary tumors, medications known to stimulate PRL release, hypothyroidism (when excessive TRH stimulates both TSH and prolactin), or idiopathic. Causes of hyperprolactinemia are shown in Table 2–4. As many as 40% of PRL producing tumors are hormonally "silent." Excess PRL inhibits

Table 2–4. Causes of Elevated Prolactin

Medications
  phenothiazines, metoclopramide,
  tricyclic antidepressants, estrogens, cimetidine
  alpha-methyl dopa, reserpine, opiates
Primary hypothyroidism
Chronic renal failure
Breast stimulation or trauma
"Empty sella" syndrome
Stress
Idiopathic
Pituitary adenomas
  microadenoma (with amenorrhea and galactorrhea)
  macroadenoma secreting prolactin
  "pseudoprolactinoma"

release of LH and FSH from the pituitary, leading to decreased stimulation of the gonads to produce sex hormones.

Clinical Presentation

The clinical syndrome most commonly associated with elevated PRL is amenorrhea and galactorrhea in women. PRL excess also occurs in males, where it presents as impotence and infertility with signs of hypogonadism, less often with gynecomastia and galactorrhea. PRL should be measured in all women with amenorrhea and in males with hypogonadotropic hypogonadism. Since excessive PRL may be clinically "silent," PRL should be measured in all patients with a pituitary mass lesion; marked prolactin excess may not be accompanied by galactorrhea. Galactorrhea may occur in the absence of abnormal prolactin secretion, and PRL measurement is not necessary if galactorrhea is minimal and menses are regular.

Diagnosis of Hyperprolactinemia

Careful history (to rule out medications that may elevate PRL, Table 2–4), TSH measurement (to rule out primary hypothyroidism, which may elevate PRL), basal PRL measurement, and CT or MRI of the pituitary all should be done in a patient suspected of having a prolactin-secreting microadenoma. Most patients with PRL levels >150 ng/mL have PRL-secreting tumors; many large prolactinomas are associated with PRL levels >1000 ng/mL. Stimulation and suppression testing have not proved useful in differentiating hyperprolactinemia due to a pituitary microadenoma from other causes. While most patients with prolactinomas fail to show an increase in PRL after TRH, the same is true for most patients with hyperprolactinemia from other causes. Unless a pituitary tumor can be demonstrated by CT or MRI, the diagnosis is one of exclusion. Since 50% of prolactinomas are too small to be seen by neuroradiologic techniques, the distinction among tumor, PRL-cell hyperplasia, and idiopathic hyperprolactinemia may not be possible short of surgery.

Simply finding an elevated PRL in a patient with a pituitary tumor does not establish a cause and effect relationship. "Pseudoprolactinomas" are large nonsecretory tumors that press on the pituitary stalk and disrupt the normal inhibitory flow of dopamine from the hypothalamus, resulting in a modest elevation in PRL. It is particularly important to make this distinction when deciding on treatment, since prolactinomas usually decrease in size with medical therapy but "pseudoprolactinomas" do not (even though prolactin levels usually come down with bromocriptine, "pseudoprolactinomas" often continue to grow). In patients with pituitary macroadenomas (≥10 mm diameter), PRL <500 ng/mL usually indicates a "pseudoprolactinoma," PRL >1000 ng/mL a true PRL-producing tumor, and values between 500 and 1000 ng/mL must be interpreted based on individual circumstances.

Treatment of Hyperprolactinemia

The natural history of *prolactin-secreting microadenomas* and *idiopathic hyperprolactinemia* in most patients is not progressive. There is rarely significant growth of tumor, but hyperprolactinemia and disordered reproductive function usually persist. When these conditions began to be recognized with increased frequency in the early 1970s, three camps of management arose: surgical, medical, and observation. (Radiation treatment is felt by most authorities to have unacceptable morbidity for these patients.) Surgical treatment has a high initial cure rate for microadenomas (85%) but recurrent hyperprolactinemia is seen in over half the early responders within 5 years of surgery. Observation may seem an appealing choice, particularly if fertility is not desired. Most of these patients are women in their 20s and 30s, and hyperprolactinemia leads to hypogonadism that is reversible with treatment; reduced bone mineral content has been shown in hyperprolactinemic women, and osteoporosis is a likely result of prolonged hypogonadism. Since estrogen has been shown to stimulate growth of prolactin-secreting cells in vitro, estrogens should be given with caution or preferably withheld. Medical treatment (bromocriptine) seems best for most of these patients, though treatment should be individualized. Neuroradiologic studies of the pituitary (CT or MRI) should be repeated 1 or 2 years after the initial evaluation to be sure that there is no tumor growth.

Bromocriptine, an orally administered dopamine agonist drug, is safe, generally well-tolerated, and usually effective in lowering serum prolactin regardless of the cause of prolactin elevation. It is also effective in reducing the size of PRL-secreting tumors, sometimes shrinking massive tumors away to nothing. For this reason, medical treatment is the first line treatment for most patients with pathologic hyperprolactinemia. There are several caveats regarding bromocriptine treatment:
   1. Many patients experience troublesome side effects (nausea, dizziness) when first starting the drug ("first dose" effects). These can be minimized by starting the first three

23

or four doses with a low dose (1.25 mg) given immediately before retiring at night.

2. There is a wide range of response to this drug. Many women have a good response to a low, single dose (1.25 or 2.5 mg/day), while others require higher or divided doses. Titrate the dose up gradually to find the minimum effective dose.

3. Treat the patient, not the test; if regular, ovulatory menses are occurring, don't be concerned about a mild or moderate prolactin elevation.

4. With idiopathic hyperprolactinemia or prolactin-secreting microadenomas, remissions are uncommon but do occur (2 to 3%). While medication must be continued lifelong in most patients, it is worth stopping after 6 months or a year to see if a remission has occurred.

5. Although no evidence exists that bromocriptine causes birth defects, there is no reason to continue it through pregnancy, either; growth of small tumors during pregnancy is unusual (less than 2% of cases). Stop the medication as soon as pregnancy is confirmed.

6. Medically-induced shrinkage of a large tumor that has eroded the sellar floor into the sphenoid sinus may lead to a CSF leak.

7. "Pseudoprolactinomas" (large, nonsecretory tumors associated with a mild or moderate increase in prolactin) often continue to grow despite a lowering of prolactin with medical treatment.

Prolactin-secreting macroadenomas (>1.0 cm) represent a much more serious disorder. Observation is not an acceptable choice; visual field defects and/or hormone deficiencies are often present at diagnosis. Surgical treatment is effective in correcting the elevated prolactin and restoring normal reproductive function in fewer than half the patients with large prolactin secreting tumors, but should be considered as an initial step in patients when vision is threatened or if medical treatment fails to show a prompt reduction in tumor size. Radiation therapy should be used as an adjunct to medical or surgical treatment; at best, prevention of tumor growth, not shrinkage, should be expected from radiation. Medical treatment is surprisingly effective in many patients with large prolactin-secreting tumors, shrinking massive tumors in 80 to 90% of patients and preserving or restoring secretion of other hormones.

Management of these patients is probably best left to major centers with substantial experience.

Bevan JS, Burke CW, Esiri MM, et al.: Misinterpretation of prolactin levels leading to management errors in patients with sellar enlargement. Am J Med 1987; *82*:29–32.

Johnston DG, Prescott RWG, Kendall-Taylor P, et al.: Hyperprolactinemia: long-term effects of bromocriptine. Am J Med 1983; *75*:868–874.

Martin TL, Kim M, Malarkey WB: The natural history of idiopathic hyperprolactinemia. J Clin Endocrinol Metab 1985; *60*:855–858.

Molitch ME: Pregnancy and the hyperprolactinemic woman. N Engl J Med 1983; *312*:1364–1370.

Molitch ME, Elton RL, Blackwell RE, et al.: Bromocriptine as primary therapy for prolactin-secreting macroadenomas: results of a prospective multicenter study. J Clin Endocrinol Metab 1985; *60*:698–705.

Schlechte JA, Sherman BM, Chapler FK, et al.: Long term follow-up of women with surgically treated prolactin-secreting pituitary tumors. J Clin Endocrinol Metab 1986; *62*:1296–1301.

Vance ML, Evans WS, Thorne MO: Bromocriptine. Ann Intern Med 1984; *100*:78–91.

Wollesen F, Bendsen BB: Effect rates of different modalities for treatment of prolactin adenomas. Am J Med 1985; *78*:114–122.

GROWTH HORMONE

Normal secretion of GH is episodic, with several peaks during a 24-hour period, particularly after stress or exercise and an hour or so after the onset of deep sleep. Increases in plasma glucose normally cause a decrease in GH and hypoglycemia stimulates a rise of GH.

The effects of GH on cartilage and possibly other tissues occur through the generation of another group of hormones, the somatomedins. These hormones are produced by the liver in response to GH. The most important of these compounds is *somatomedin-C,* also known as insulin-like growth factor-1 (IGF-1). Somatomedins stimulate uptake of sulfate by cartilage and were first called "sulfation factor." Their effects are more general, however, and include increased synthesis of collagen and proteoglycans, inhibition of lipolysis, and other metabolic effects such as positive balances of nitrogen, phosphorus, potassium, magnesium, and calcium, and an increase in protein synthesis. GH has divergent effects on carbohydrate metabolism; initially, an injection of GH causes a fall in blood glucose; chronic GH excess inhibits glucose entry into cells, antagonistic to the action of insulin. This leads to glucose intolerance and in some cases, overt diabetes.

GH DEFICIENCY

GH deficiency is the most common pituitary hormone deficiency state but is clinically significant only in children, when it results in short stature.

Background, Pathophysiology

Normal growth is the result of the interaction of multiple hormones and systems, of which growth hormone is only one. GH deficiency as an isolated defect is often due to deficient production of GHRH by the hypothalamus, but GH deficiency alone or in combination with other hormone deficiencies may also result from pituitary or hypothalamic tumors, such as craniopharyngioma. GH deficiency must be differentiated from other causes of short stature.

Clinical Presentation

Growth retardation in severe GH deficiency may be apparent by 6 months of age; when the deficiency is mild, the onset of growth delay will be later. In addition to short stature, children with growth hormone deficiency are often mildly obese (growth hormone is lipolytic, and its absence favors accumulation of adipose tissue).

Diagnosis of GH Deficiency

To test for GH reserve, provocative agents such as insulin (protocol p. 214), L-dopa (protocol, p. 215) arginine, and glucagon can be given; brisk exercise is a simple nonpharmacologic stimulus for GH release. None of these agents is infallible; failure of GH to increase after two of these agents is highly suspicious for GH deficiency, but 20% of normal individuals will fail to respond to one of these agents on a single occasion. Also, some patients with partial GH deficiency respond to these provocative agents but show a diminished magnitude and number of GH secretory episodes during the day. In most centers, the diagnosis of GH deficiency is based on a reduced magnitude or number of GH secretory episodes in multiple samples obtained during a 24-hour period.

Somatomedin-C levels are usually low in children with GH deficiency, and somatomedin-C measurement is a good screening test for GH deficiency (it has a longer half-life than GH) (Fig. 2–3). However, levels of somatomedin-C may be low in other causes of growth failure, and some children with normal levels of somatomedin-C will show accelerated growth if treated

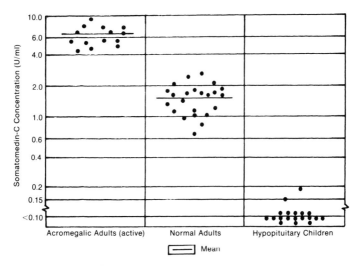

Fig. 2–3. Somatomedin levels. (Used with permission; illustration by Albert Miller, from Furlanetto RW et al, J Clin Invest 1977; *60*:648, *in* VanWyk JJ, Underwood LE. Growth hormone, somatomedins, and growth failure. Hosp Practice 1978; *13*:57–67.)

with GH. Evaluation of children with severe short stature or who are otherwise highly suspect for having GH deficiency is probably best done in a referral center.

Treatment of GH Deficiency

Biosynthetic human GH is now available and is clearly effective in promoting growth in GH deficient subjects. The usual dose is 0.1 mg/kg intramuscularly three times a week. Until recently, GH for treatment was extracted from human pituitary glands and was in limited supply. It was removed from the market in 1985 because of presumed contamination of some lots with slow virus (Creutzfeldt-Jakob disease). Biosynthetic GH is expensive, but now that availability is no longer limited there is speculation that it will be used to increase final height in short but otherwise normal children. Efficacy and safety in this regard are not yet established; at present, it seems appropriate to reserve GH treatment for children with established GH deficiency or as part of a research protocol.

Growth hormone releasing-hormone (GHRH) given by a portable infusion pump has been shown to stimulate release of endogenous growth hormone and stimulate growth in children with GH deficiency due to hypothalamic dysfunction. GHRH

27

is a much smaller molecule than GH and thus should be easier to synthesize and ultimately be cheaper.

Bercu BB, Shulman D, Root AW, et al.: Growth hormone (GH) provocative testing frequently does not reflect endogenous GH secretion. J Clin Endocrinol Metab 1986; *63*:709–716.

Biosynthetic growth hormone. Med Lett Drugs Therap 1985; *27*:101–102.

(Editorial) Who needs growth hormone? Lancet 1984; *2*:1189–1190.

Grossman A, Savage MO, Wass JAH, et al.: Growth-hormone-releasing factor in growth hormone deficiency: demonstration of a hypothalamic defect in growth hormone release. Lancet 1983; *2*:137–138.

Rechler MM, Nissley SP, Roth J: Hormonal regulation of human growth. N Engl J Med 1987; *316*:941–942.

Spiliotis BE, August GP, Hung W, et al.: Growth hormone neurosecretory dysfunction: a treatable cause of short stature. JAMA 1984; *251*:2223–2230.

Underwood LE: Report of the conference on uses and possible abuses of biosynthetic human growth hormone. N Engl J Med 1984; *311*:606–608.

Vance ML, Thorner MO: Growth-hormone-releasing hormone: a clinical update. Ann Intern Med 1986; *105*:447–449.

ACROMEGALY

Background, Pathophysiology

Chronic hypersecretion of growth hormone (GH), usually by a pituitary adenoma, leads to the syndrome of acromegaly in adults and to pituitary gigantism in children. Acromegaly is an uncommon condition but accounts for approximately 10% of all pituitary tumors. It usually occurs in the middle decades of life, though it can occur at any age. The incidence of acromegaly is estimated at 3 cases per million population, and the prevalence is approximately 40 per million. Pituitary gigantism is quite rare.

Most patients with acromegaly or pituitary gigantism have a pituitary tumor shown by CT scan or found at surgery. The character of these tumors is variable. Most contain secretory granules by electron microscopy that can be shown by immunoperoxidase staining to contain GH. On light microscopy the granules usually stain eosinophilic (or acidophilic) with H&E, but sometimes they do not stain (chromophobic). Up to one third of GH secreting tumors also appear to secrete prolactin.

It is not known whether these tumors arise as the result of a primary disorder in the pituitary gland or from a defect in the hypothalamus that leads secondarily to the pituitary tumor, such as an excess of growth hormone releasing hormone (GHRH). There is evidence for and against both possibilities. Rare causes of acromegaly include ectopic production of GHRH (by pancreatic or other tumors) and, in at least one case, ectopic production of GH (by a pancreatic neoplasm).

Many aspects of GH dynamics are abnormal in acromegaly. GH secretion is sustained in some patients but episodic in others, sometimes with widely fluctuating levels. Even when GH is only slightly elevated, oral glucose does not show the usual suppressive effect. Many patients with acromegaly have a decrease in GH after administration of the dopamine agonist drug bromocriptine, an agent that does not affect GH secretion in normal subjects.

Approximately 50% of patients with acromegaly show an increase in GH after thyrotropin releasing hormone (TRH), and 50% respond to gonadotropin releasing hormone (GnRH) with an increase in GH. Demonstration of these abnormal dynamic responses is useful in the patient whose post-glucose GH value is not diagnostically elevated. From the perspective of clinical research, investigating these abnormal responses provides further knowledge regarding etiology, pathophysiology, and response to treatment.

Chronic hypersecretion of GH, through increased production of somatomedins, leads to the recognizable increases in growth of soft tissues, cartilage, and bone that are characteristic of acromegaly. Thickening of the skin is due to interstitial edema, deposits of hyaluronates, and increased connective tissue. The metabolic changes of acromegaly result from the actions of GH on fuel and mineral metabolism.

Clinical Presentation

Since acromegaly may be insidious and subtle, a high degree of clinical suspicion is needed to make an early diagnosis. Changing facial features or increasing shoe, ring, or hat size would warrant further consideration, and the diagnosis should be entertained in any patient with unexplained neuropathy or puzzling rheumatic symptoms. Pituitary gigantism is rare, but should be suspected in children who show unusually rapid growth.

Family history is usually not contributory in patients with acromegaly; however, acromegaly is sometimes seen as a feature of multiple endocrine neoplasia, type I, which also includes hyperparathyroidism and islet cell tumors of the pancreas.

The symptoms of acromegaly depend on the stage of the disease. Common signs and symptoms are shown in Table 2–5. Morbidity from acromegaly occurs primarily from peripheral neuropathy (foot drop, muscle atrophy, Charcot joints), problems with the cardiovascular system (hypertension, cardiomegaly, sometimes with fulminant congestive heart failure), and mass effects from the pituitary tumor (visual field cuts or blindness, cranial nerve involvement, and hypopituitarism). Although some patients with acromegaly have a benign course and occasional spontaneous remissions occur, the overall life expectancy of patients with untreated acromegaly is reduced.

Abnormalities found in routine studies may include hyperglycemia and glycosuria; serum phosphorus is often elevated. While urinary calcium excretion is frequently increased, serum calcium is usually normal. Evidence of cardiomegaly may be seen on chest x ray or electrocardiogram.

Diagnosis of Acromegaly

Patients with active acromegaly have abnormal dynamics of GH secretion. A simple diagnostic approach is to measure serum GH one hour after the oral administration of 100 g of glucose (protocol, p. 212). Clearly elevated GH level (>10 ng/mL) after oral glucose, combined with the clinical picture, makes the diagnosis of acromegaly secure, while a normal level of GH after oral glucose (<5 ng/mL) essentially rules out the diagnosis. Only a small percentage of subjects being investigated for acromegaly will have a post-glucose GH level that is intermediate (5 to 10 ng/mL). In these patients, other tests can be used to define their status. Measurements of somatomedin-C reflect the

Table 2–5. **Signs and Symptoms of Acromegaly**

Coarsening of facial features
Enlargement of hands, feet, and jaw
Headache
Evidence of peripheral neuropathy
Carpal tunnel and other compartment syndromes
Muscle weakness
Joint pain and stiffness (degenerative joint disease)
Visual field defects
Skin changes:
    thickening, coarseness
    increased sweating
Hirsutism
Endocrine changes:
    galactorrhea
    menstrual disturbances, decreased libido
    goiter (with or without thyroid dysfunction)

---

integrated production of GH, and serve as a useful confirmatory adjunct to GH measurements or as a screening test to "rule out" acromegaly (Fig. 2–3).

Though computed tomography (CT) or magnetic resonance (MR) imaging will often show a pituitary tumor in patients with acromegaly, these anatomic tests should be deferred until biochemical evidence of GH excess has been established. In the rare cases where ectopic production of GHRH has been the cause of acromegaly, abdominal GHRH-producing tumors have been detected by CT scanning.

Treatment of Acromegaly

In most cases of acromegaly, *transsphenoidal surgery* and selective tumor removal is the treatment of choice. In experienced hands, this operation offers the best chance for cure (44 to 90% in reported series; chance of cure is best with smaller tumors), and has low morbidity and mortality; anterior pituitary function is usually preserved.

Two types of *radiation therapy* have been used to treat acromegaly—conventional (e.g., cobalt) and heavy particle irradiation. Conventional irradiation leads to a reduction of GH and clinical improvement in 70 to 80% of patients; however, radiation requires a relatively long time before the beneficial effects are seen (often 2 to 4 years), and more importantly, there are serious delayed risks of radiation including hypopituitarism, cataracts, optic nerve damage, and CNS tumors. Conventional radiation should be reserved for patients with surgically incurable or recurrent tumors or when surgery cannot be performed. Heavy particle irradiation (e.g., proton beam therapy) can provide good control of acromegaly with an acceptable incidence of side effects, but this therapeutic modality is not used as much currently as it was 10 to 12 years ago because of the increasing use of transsphenoidal surgery and concerns over the long-term effects of high doses of radiation. Also, heavy particle therapy requires specialized equipment that is available in only two centers in the U.S.

Medical treatment of acromegaly has not been generally successful. Over the years, a number of drugs have been used, including chlorpromazine, estrogens, and antiserotonin agents. The most effective and practical drugs currently in use are dopamine agonists such as bromocriptine. Bromocriptine lowers serum GH in up to 75% of patients, but in only 20% are the levels reduced to normal; patients in whom prolactin is elevated are more likely to have a favorable response. The dose of bromocriptine in acromegaly ranges from 15 to 50 mg/day. Continuous treatment is required, as withdrawal of the drug is associated with a prompt return of elevated serum GH levels. In contrast to prolactinomas, GH-secreting tumors do not usually decrease in size with bromocriptine. Bromocriptine has an adjunctive role in patients who fail to achieve a cure by surgical treatment or who are to be treated with radiation. Not yet released for general use but promising in early trials, a long-acting *analog of somatostatin* appears quite effective and safe for treatment of acromegaly, even in patients who have not responded to surgery or radiation. Patients with an incomplete response to the somatostatin analog often do well with the addition of bromocriptine. With further experience, long-term treatment with this somatostatin analog may well merit consideration as first-line treatment of acromegaly.

Periodic reassessment of GH production is advisable after treatment, particularly soon after surgery. Criteria for cure are a normal basal GH level and normal GH dynamic responses. If the basal GH is <2 ng/mL, normal dynamics can be assumed; if the basal GH is >10 ng/mL, abnormal dynamics are almost certain. Patients with intermediate GH levels should be tested further with oral glucose suppression or with stimulation tests using TRH, GnRH, or both. Somatomedin-C levels appear to correlate better with clinical activity than GH levels do and should be followed. Patients should be carefully followed for enlargement or recurrence of a pituitary mass lesion (including CT or MR scans of the sella and visual field determinations).

Barnard LB, Grantham WG, Lamberton P, et al.: Treatment of resistant acromegaly with a long-acting somatostatin analogue (SMS 201–995). Ann Intern Med 1986; *105*:856–861.

Clemmons DR, Van Wyk JJ, Ridgeway EC, et al.: Evaluation of acromegaly by radioimmunoassay of somatomedin-C. N Engl J Med 1979; *301*:1138–1142.

Earll JM, Sparks LL, Forsham PH: Glucose suppression of serum growth hormone in the diagnosis of acromegaly. JAMA 1967; *201*:134–136.

Jadresic A: Recent developments in acromegaly: a review. J Royal Soc Med 1983; *76*:947–956.

Lamberts SWJ, Zweens M, Verschoor L, et al.: A comparison among growth hormone-lowering effects in acromegaly of the somatostatin analog SMS 201–995, bromocriptine, and the combination of both drugs. J Clin Endocrinol Metab 1986; *63*:16–19.

Melmed S, Braunstein EH, Ezrin C, et al.: Pathophysiology of acromegaly. Endocr Rev 1983; *4*:271–290.

Pearson OH, Arafah B, Brodkey J: Management of acromegaly. Ann Intern Med 1981; *95*:225–227.

Serri O, Somma M, Comtois R, et al.: Acromegaly: biochemical assessment of cure after long term follow-up of transsphenoidal selective adenomectomy. J Clin Endocrinol Metab 1985; *61*:1185–1189.

LESS COMMON PITUITARY CONDITIONS

Thyroid Stimulating Hormone

TSH deficiency due to pituitary or hypothalamic disease leads to hypothyroidism (called secondary or tertiary hypothyroidism), though hypothyroidism is most commonly due to thyroid gland failure (primary hypothyroidism). TSH deficiency is rarely seen as an isolated finding, but commonly accompanies other hormone deficiencies in patients who have large tumors of the pituitary or hypothalamus. Severe illness causes changes in the hypothalamic-pituitary-thyroid axis that may be difficult to differentiate from hypothalamic or pituitary disease ("euthyroid sick syndrome"); it appears that the pituitary and/or hypothalamus lower their level of response during severe chronic illness so that lower levels of thyroid hormone can be maintained.

Excessive autonomous production of TSH is rare. When it is the result of a pituitary tumor, it leads to hyperthyroidism. Overproduction of TSH also occurs in states of tissue resistance to thyroid hormone, also rare. The most common cause of TSH elevation is thyroid gland failure, even in the earliest stages. If hypothyroidism is long-standing and severe, it may lead to pituitary enlargement and may be confused with a pituitary adenoma. In these cases, treatment of hypothyroidism causes resolution of the pituitary enlargement.

Adrenocorticotropic Hormone

ACTH deficiency results in cortisol deficiency and the syndrome of adrenal insufficiency, with signs and symptoms that include weakness, weight loss, nausea and vomiting, and hypotension. Primary failure of the adrenal glands (Addison's disease) results in deficiency of mineralocorticoids as well as cortisol, and is much more frequent than secondary failure (pituitary or hypothalamic disease). ACTH deficiency is usually due to pituitary or hypothalamic tumors, but is rarely seen as an isolated finding.

When ACTH secretion is diminished, the adrenal glands rapidly become atrophic, so direct testing of cortisol production is a good index of the hypothalamic-pituitary-adrenal axis. Cortisol production can be assessed by measuring AM serum cortisol, or by a simple stimulation test, giving an injection of the biologically active fragment of ACTH (cosyntropin, 250 μg IV or IM) and looking for a normal increase in plasma cortisol (protocol, p. 207). A normal response (rise in serum cortisol >7 μg/dL and peak value >18 μg/dL) makes any form of adrenal insufficiency highly unlikely. Failure to increase cortisol in this test is always seen in primary adrenal disease and usually in pituitary or hypothalamic disease causing ACTH deficiency. If there is a subnormal cortisol rise after cosyntropin, plasma ACTH can be measured; a high value points to primary adrenal disease, while a low or "normal" level in the face of low adrenal function indicates pituitary or hypothalamic disease.

Levels of ACTH are not usually measured in stimulation or suppression tests, in part because the simpler assays of adrenal response usually provide the necessary information, and partly because of technical difficulties with the ACTH assay. For ACTH measurements, blood should be drawn in heparinized tubes, promptly chilled in ice water, and stored in plastic vials until assayed.

Standard tests of pituitary ACTH reserve include the insulin tolerance test (ITT) (protocol, p. 214) and metyrapone test (protocol, p. 216). These tests are generally reserved for situations where simpler tests have failed to provide satisfactory information. The stress of insulin-induced hypoglycemia leads to the release of ACTH; measuring the increase of cortisol that results is the usual end point. This test is potentially risky and is usually performed in the hospital. An alternate test involves the administration of metyrapone, a drug that partially inhibits cortisol production; the fall in cortisol leads to a rise in ACTH which drives the adrenal glands to overcome this block, resulting in an increase in the steroid compound that immediately precedes cortisol–11-deoxycortisol (compound S)–which can be measured directly in blood, or in urine as 17-hydroxysteroids. Neither of these tests can invariably differentiate hypothalamic from pituitary disease. Recently, corticotropin releasing hormone (CRH) has become available for testing. In normal subjects, CRH stimulates a brisk rise of ACTH and secondarily, a rise in cortisol. It is likely that this agent will largely replace the other tests of pituitary ACTH reserve.

Excessive production of ACTH leads to overproduction of cortisol by the adrenal glands, resulting in the striking clinical picture of Cushing's syndrome, which is discussed at length in the section on adrenal diseases. *Nelson's syndrome* is the presence of an aggressive ACTH-secreting pituitary tumor and occurs in up to 30% of patients with pituitary Cushing's disease who are treated with bilateral adrenalectomy. Hyperpigmentation is a striking feature and is due to MSH activity associated with the high ACTH level. Since the current treatment of choice in pituitary Cushing's is transsphenoidal surgery to remove the pituitary tumor, Nelson's syndrome is seen much less often now than in the past.

Gonadotropins (Follicle Stimulating Hormone and Luteinizing Hormone)

Deficient production of gonadotropins leads to hypogonadism. Deficiencies of LH and FSH usually occur together, and may be due to destructive or infiltrating lesions of the pituitary and/or hypothalamus, the inhibitory effect of excessive PRL on gonadotropin release, or central problems such as anorexia nervosa, stress, weight loss, or intense physical training. Congenital deficiency of gonadotropins occurs and becomes apparent when puberty fails to occur on schedule. Gonadotropin measurements are quite useful in evaluating abnormalities of pubertal development or gonadal function. In patients with hypogonadism, elevations of LH and FSH indicate a primary gonadal problem, while low or "normal" values point to a pituitary or hypothalamic defect. Stimulation tests with GnRH or clomiphene (an antiestrogen that blocks negative feedback on the pituitary, normally causing a rise of LH and FSH) have not proved consistently reliable or superior to basal measurements. Since secretion of LH and FSH is pulsatile, measurement of gonadotropins in urine, which provides a more "integrated" picture, may be preferred in some situations to measurements in blood.

Excessive secretion of LH and FSH by pituitary tumors is quite rare. Nearly all of the reported cases have been large tumors. In polycystic ovary syndrome and other hyperandrogenic states, LH is increased but FSH is normal. It is not known whether this change is a primary factor or secondary to the androgen excess.

Empty Sella Syndrome

The primary "empty sella" syndrome refers to a patient with an enlarged pituitary fossa that partially contains cerebral spinal fluid, presumably due to an anatomic abnormality or increased CSF pressure or both. Most patients with this condition are obese middle-aged females. The enlarged sella may be dis-

35

covered accidentally; complaints that may be related include headache, other signs and symptoms related to increased intracranial pressure, and variable degrees of anterior pituitary insufficiency. An "empty sella" may also be acquired secondary to trauma or infarction. Evaluation of TSH, ACTH, and gonadotropins should be done in these patients. Prolactin is occasionally elevated. This disorder is usually not progressive and does not usually require treatment. It can often be differentiated from space-occupying lesions by high-resolution CT scanning with or without metrizamide (a contrast material that can be introduced into the CSF to outline the CSF space).

Pituitary Apoplexy

This condition is a neurologic catastrophe. Patients may have no previous symptoms or be known to have a pre-existing pituitary adenoma. There is sudden onset of symptoms including some or all of the following: nausea, vomiting, severe headache, photophobia, decreased vision, diplopia, and altered consciousness. This condition results from acute hemorrhage into a pituitary tumor and requires emergency neurosurgical decompression. Patients should be presumed to have adrenal insufficiency and covered with stress doses of hydrocortisone until their condition permits adequate endocrine testing.

Jaffer KA, Obbens EA, El-Gammalf TA: "Empty" sella: review of 76 cases. South Med J 1979; 72:294–296.

Klibanski A, Deutsch PJ, Jameson JL, et al.: Luteinizing hormone-secreting pituitary tumor: biosynthetic characterization and clinical studies. J Clin Endocrinol Metab 1987; 64:536–543.

Weintraub BD, Gershengorn MC, Kourides IA, et al.: Inappropriate secretion of thyroid-stimulating hormone. Ann Intern Med 1981; 95:339–351.

Posterior Pituitary, Hyponatremia

THE POSTERIOR PITUITARY; POLYURIC DISORDERS; HYPONATREMIA

The posterior lobe of the pituitary gland consists of nerve fibers that store the two hormones that are produced in the supraoptic and paraventricular nuclei of the hypothalamus. *Oxytocin* is released in response to suckling and serves to stimulate lactation and uterine contractions. The other hormone of the posterior pituitary, *antidiuretic hormone* (ADH) or *vasopressin* is involved with regulation of water balance. ADH is the only one of these hormones of general clinical significance. The focus of this chapter will be on the diagnosis and treatment of ADH deficiency (diabetes insipidus) and ADH excess (syndrome of inappropriate ADH secretion—SIADH). Commonly encountered clinical conditions that must be considered in the differential diagnosis will be mentioned; for complete discussion of uncommon conditions such as "reset osmostat" or abnormalities of thirst, a standard textbook of endocrinology should be consulted.

Background, Pathophysiology

The principal stimulus for ADH release is an increase in serum osmolality; other important stimuli include a decrease in effective plasma volume or arterial pressure, pain, stress, sleep, exercise, and drugs such as nicotine, morphine, and barbiturates. ADH release is inhibited by reduced serum osmolality, elevated arterial blood pressure, exposure to cold, alcohol, and drugs including phenytoin and glucocorticoids.

ADH directly regulates water reabsorption from the distal renal tubule, indirectly controlling the concentration of osmotically active solutes (such as sodium) in the extracellular fluid. In addition, ADH in large concentrations induces vasoconstriction and a rise in arterial pressure (thus the alternate name, vasopressin).

HANDY CALCULATIONS

Osmolality in serum or plasma may be estimated for most clinical purposes as twice the sum of sodium and potassium concentrations. A more accurate way to calculate serum osmolality is the formula:

$2([Na^+] + [K^+]) + (BUN/2.8) + (glucose/18)$

Body water and its compartments may be estimated:
total body water (TBW) in liters = wt (kg) × 0.6
intracellular fluid (ICF) in liters = wt (kg) × 0.4
extracellular fluid (ECF) in liters = wt (kg) × 0.2

Pseudohyponatremia refers to a spurious lowering of serum sodium either by an increase in another osmotically active substance (such as glucose or protein) leading to a shift of water from ICF to ECF, or an increase in the lipid content of serum that partitions with the aqueous phase. The "corrected" serum sodium may be determined by adding the following amounts to the measured serum sodium level:
glucose excess (mg/dL) × 0.016
lipids (mg/dL) × 0.002
protein excess (g/dL) × 0.25

For further reading on basic concepts in hyper- and hyponatremia, the following article is recommended: Rose BD: New approach to disturbances in the plasma sodium concentration. Am J Med 1986; *81*:1033–1040.

DIABETES INSIPIDUS (DI)

Clinical Presentation

Patients with deficient production or action of ADH have polyuria, since the renal tubule is unable to reabsorb solute-free water in the absence of ADH. Urine output >2.5 L/d should be considered abnormal and investigated further; with complete ADH deficiency, urine output may reach 1 L/h. The differential diagnosis of polyuria includes deficient ADH production (central DI), decreased ADH action on the kidney (nephrogenic DI), and excessive water drinking (psychogenic polydipsia). In DI, when thirst is normal and access to water is unlimited, serum osmolality and electrolytes will usually remain normal; urinary water loss in excess of intake leads to hypernatremia and dehydration.

ADH deficiency (central DI) may be idiopathic or due to destructive or infiltrative lesions of the hypothalamus or pituitary; central DI is a common (but usually transient) complication of pituitary surgery. Central DI may be partial or complete. Nephrogenic DI may result from conditions affecting the kidney including amyloidosis, multiple myeloma, chronic electrolyte abnormalities (hypokalemia or hypercalcemia), and medications such as lithium, demeclocycline, and methoxyflurane. Nephrogenic DI may be idiopathic or inherited, partial or complete, transient or permanent.

Diagnosis of Diabetes Insipidus

First, polyuria should be documented. Most out-patients can measure their urine output for 24 hours and report the volume. If desired, creatinine content of the collection can be measured as an estimate of completeness; alcohol, nicotine, and caffeine should be avoided. If polyuria is confirmed and common causes such as diabetes mellitus excluded, further investigation should be done in the hospital, particularly if polyuria is severe; many of these patients will experience substantial fluid loss and dehydration during diagnostic maneuvers. A recommended approach to the diagnosis and differential diagnosis of polyuric states is shown in Table 3–1.

The classic diagnostic strategy for diabetes insipidus is the water deprivation test (protocol, p. 219). If access to water is denied, patients with central or nephrogenic DI cannot conserve free water and show weight loss, hypernatremia, and an increase of plasma osmolality; urine osmolality remains low, typically less than plasma. Once urine osmolality has stabilized, administration of vasopressin will distinguish central DI (where

Table 3–1. Diagnosis of Diabetes Insipidus

Document polyuria (urine volume ≥2.5 L/d) and exclude glycosuria

If plasma osmolality is ≥295 mOsm/kg or serum sodium ≥145 mEq/L, primary polydipsia is unlikely; proceed with overnight water deprivation test (protocol, p. 219) or hypertonic saline infusion (protocol, p. 217).

Overnight water deprivation test: if the ratio of urine to plasma osmolality is <1.5 at the end of the test, primary polydipsia is unlikely. Measure plasma and urine osmolality and plasma ADH at the end of the test; use these relationships to differentiate normal, nephrogenic or central DI, and psychogenic polydipsia. If urine osmolality is ≤400 mOsm/kg at end of test, give 5 U of aqueous vasopressin SQ. If urine osmolality increases ≥10%, central diabetes insipidus is probable; if urine osmolality does not increase, nephrogenic diabetes insipidus is highly probable.

Hypertonic saline infusion: plot plasma osmolality vs. plasma ADH (see Fig. 3–1).

(Used with permission from Chattoraj SC, Watts NB: *in* Tietz NW (ed): Textbook of Clinical Chemistry, 2nd ed. Philadelphia, WB Saunders, 1986, p. 1035.)

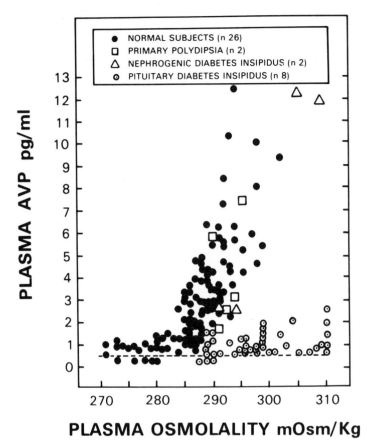

Fig. 3–1. The relationship of plasma AVP (ADH) to plasma osmolality in normal and polyuric subjects. (Reproduced from The Journal of Clinical Investigation, 1973; *52*:2340–2352 by copyright permission of the American Society for Clinical Investigation; Robertson GL, Mahr EA, Athar S, Sinha T: Development and clinical application of a new method for the radioimmunoassay of arginine vasopressin in human plasma.)

urine osmolality increases >10% after vasopressin) from nephrogenic DI (no response to vasopressin). Most patients with psychogenic polydipsia have a normal urine osmolality after water deprivation, but some of these patients fail to produce a concentrated urine unless water deprivation is prolonged (presumably from "wash-out" of solutes from the renal medulla, which interferes with maximal urine concentrating ability).

Measurement of ADH in serum is now available from several reference labs. After water deprivation, when serum osmolality is increased, patients with central DI have low or inappropriately "normal" ADH levels, while patients with nephrogenic

DI have high plasma ADH. Since ADH levels discriminate best when the patient is hyperosmolal, ADH can be measured after hypertonic saline solution is given to produce a hyperosmolal state (protocol, p. 217) if results after water deprivation are inconclusive.

Treatment of Diabetes Insipidus

Complete central DI (urine volumes >10 L/d) usually requires administration of some form of vasopressin. Of course, fluid and electrolyte abnormalities that result from excess water loss should be corrected. Several forms of vasopressin are available.

1. *DDAVP* (des-amino, D-arginine vasopressin), a chemical modification of the ADH molecule with prolonged action and little pressor activity, can be given intranasally or parenterally, and is the most satisfactory preparation for long term use. Most patients can be managed with 0.1 to 0.2 mL intranasally once or twice a day. The dose should be titrated based on urine output and serum sodium levels. In addition to treatment of DI, parenteral DDAVP is used to increase levels of clotting factor VIII in classic hemophilia!

2. *Aqueous vasopressin* is given parenterally (IM or SQ; usual dose 5 U every 4 to 8 h). It is less expensive than parenteral DDAVP and for this reason, usually the preparation of choice when short-term parenteral treatment is required. It is shorter acting than DDAVP and has more pressor activity; the latter property may present a problem when using this preparation to treat patients who have elevated or unstable arterial pressure.

3. Other analogues that are used much less commonly include *vasopressin tannate in oil,* a long-acting (18 to 36h) IM preparation; and *Diapid* (lysine-vasopressin), a nasal spray with a short (4 to 6 h) duration of action.

Patients with mild or moderate central DI may respond to treatment with a low dose of a *thiazide diuretic,* which is thought to work by decreasing sodium delivery to the distal tubule and thus diminish free water excretion. The oral hypoglycemic agent *chlorpropamide* (125 to 250 mg/d) and the lipid-lowering agent *clofibrate* (500 mg QID) appear to stimulate ADH release and to sensitize the renal tubular cells to low concentrations of ADH. For patients with nephrogenic DI, where the kidney is incapable of responding to ADH, thiazide diuretics may be the only effective treatment.

41

Diabetes Insipidus After Neurological Surgery

After pituitary surgery, 10 to 20% of patients experience diabetes insipidus; it is usually mild and transient, often resolving after 24 hours or less. The diagnosis is relatively straightforward: if a patient is eliminating large volumes of urine, it is either due to central DI or the appropriate excretion of previously administered fluids. It is not uncommon for patients to receive 1.5 to 2 L of fluid during surgery and to delay elimination of the extra fluid for several hours afterwards. If pulse and blood pressure are stable, the serum sodium level gives the best indication of DI (elevated if DI is present, normal or low if polyuria is due to appropriate excretion of previously administered fluid). Urine osmolality or specific gravity is not useful in this setting, being low whether the problem is DI or appropriate diuresis.

Intake and output should be measured and recorded, including fluids given during surgery and urine output during that time. For the first few days after surgery, serum sodium should be checked each morning and at any time urine output seems excessive.

Mild degrees of diabetes insipidus may not require treatment other than additional IV or PO fluids. Treatment with antidiuretic hormone should be considered in the following circumstances:

1. correction or prevention of dehydration,
2. correction or prevention of electrolyte abnormalities,
3. patient's comfort (prevention of severe thirst or urinary frequency that interferes with rest).

It seems desirable, where possible, for serum sodium and osmolality to be left slightly higher than normal to provide a stimulus for recovery of ADH production. For most patients with postoperative DI, the problem resolves in a day or two; using ADH treatment only for the above indications and only for partial correction of hypernatremia allows the determination of whether treatment will need to be continued after discharge. When ADH treatment is needed in the first few days after pituitary surgery, either short (aqueous vasopressin 5 U SQ) or intermediate (DDAVP 0.1 mL intranasally) acting preparations should be used. It is not advisable to order ADH to be given PRN based solely on urine volume; if the patient becomes slightly overhydrated after ADH administration, that excess free water will be excreted when the dose of ADH wears off, and urine output will be appropriately elevated at that time.

Miller M, Dalakos T, Moses AM, et al.: Recognition of partial defects in antidiuretic hormone secretion. Ann Intern Med 1970; *73*:721–729.

Price JDE, Lauener RW: Serum and urine osmolalities in the differential diagnosis of polyuric states. J Clin Endocrinol Metab 1966; *26*:143–148.

Robertson GL, Aycinena P, Zerbe RL: Neurogenic disorders of osmoregulation. Am J Med 1982; *72*:339–353.

Shucart WA, Jackson I: Management of diabetes insipidus in neurosurgical patients. J Neurosurg 1976; *44*:65–70.

Zerbe RL, Robertson GL: A comparison of plasma vasopressin measurements with a standard indirect test in the differential diagnosis of polyuria. N Engl J Med 1981; *305*:1539–1546.

SYNDROME OF INAPPROPRIATE ANTIDIURETIC HORMONE (SIADH)

Background, Pathophysiology

Excessive concentrations of ADH lead to retention of free water by the kidney, volume expansion, and dilutional hyponatremia. Dilutional hyponatremia may also be due to congestive heart failure, renal insufficiency, chronic liver disease, glucocorticoid deficiency, hypothyroidism, excess administration of hypotonic fluids, diuretics, and drugs that stimulate ADH (e.g., chlorpropamide). Hyponatremia may also result from depletion of total body sodium as a result of mineralocorticoid deficiency or excessive salt loss from kidney or gastrointestinal disease.

SIADH is defined as continued release of ADH in the absence of osmotic stimuli and may be due to one of several causes; production of ADH by a malignancy (such as small-cell carcinoma of the lung), central nervous system diseases (such as head injuries or strokes), or medications (such as vincristine, chlorpropamide, or carbamazepine).

Clinical Presentation

Manifestations of hyponatremia are nonspecific; these include weakness, altered consciousness (lethargy, confusion, coma), or convulsions. There are no signs or symptoms that are specific for SIADH. History, physical examination, and routine laboratory tests (BUN, creatinine, uric acid, hematocrit) often suggest that hyponatremia is dilutional or depletional.

Diagnosis of SIADH

Measurement of sodium and osmolality in plasma and urine, combined with clinical assessment of volume status, usually permit appropriate differential diagnosis of hyponatremic conditions. Typically, patients with SIADH have hypoosmolal plasma (<270 mOsm/kg), urine osmolality slightly greater than plasma (300 to 400 mOsm/kg), and urine sodium concentration that is neither high nor low (generally 40 to 80 mEq/L). Patients with excess water intake have hypotonic plasma, urine sodium >80 mEq/L, and dilute urine (urine osmolality less than plasma). Patients with hyponatremia due to sodium depletion have hypotonic plasma, low urine sodium (<20 mEq/L), and urine osmolality greater than serum (>600 mOsm/kg); patients with depletional hyponatremia due to impaired renal conservation of sodium (salt-wasting renal disease or mineralocorticoid deficiency) will have similar results except that urine sodium will be high.

If the cause of hyponatremia remains unclear with the above tests, a water loading test may be done (protocol, p. 220); patients with SIADH are unable to excrete a water load normally. The water loading test is potentially hazardous and should not be done if the serum sodium is <130 mEq/L. Plasma ADH determination is not usually needed in these patients, but would be expected to be high relative to the hypoosmolality. Table 3–2 shows a systematic approach to the diagnosis of hyponatremic disorders.

Treatment of SIADH

The cause of hyponatremia in SIADH is water excess, not sodium deificiency; thus, treatment of SIADH should be directed at elimination of free water. In mild cases, this may be achieved by simply restricting fluid intake to 1000–1500 mL/d. In more severe cases, particularly when the electrolyte abnormality is associated with seizures or other serious manifestations, correction may be obtained by giving a loop diuretic like furosemide to eliminate water and sodium, measuring the amount of sodium eliminated in the urine, then replacing the sodium lost with hypertonic (3 or 5%) sodium chloride. In an emergency situation, administration of hypertonic or isotonic saline solution without diuresis may transiently raise the serum sodium concentration in patients with SIADH; 200 to 300 mL of hypertonic saline solution can be given by rapid intravenous infusion. However, when hyponatremia is severe, correcting it

44

Table 3–2. Diagnosis of SIADH

Document plasma hypo-osmolality ($\leq$270 mOsm/kg) and hyponatremia (sodium $\leq$130 mEq/L).

Use history, physical examination, and appropriate tests to exclude cardiac, hepatic, renal, or adrenal failure or hypothyroidism (SIADH cannot be diagnosed unless these factors are corrected)

Measure urine sodium and osmolality
  Low urine sodium ($\leq$20 mEq/L) means total body sodium depletion.
  Urine osmolality less than plasma means simple water excess
  Urine osmolality greater than plasma osmolality and without correspondingly low urine sodium (usually >60 mEq/L) means SIADH is probable

If further tests seem needed:
  Water loading test (protocol p 220)—use with caution (normal results exclude SIADH).
  Measure plasma ADH and plasma renin; SIADH is characterized by hypoosmolality, high ADH, and low renin; if both are low, the problem lies with a primary defect in renal water excretion.

(Used with permission from Chattoraj SC, Watts NB: *in* Tietz NW (ed): Textbook of Clinical Chemistry, 2nd ed. Philadelphia, WB Saunders, 1986, p. 1038.)

too rapidly may lead to permanent neurologic damage, central pontine myelinolysis. Once the "crisis" has passed, further correction should proceed slowly. Since sodium concentrations above 120 mEq/L appear to be well tolerated, treatment should proceed slowly once that level has been reached.

Patients with chronic SIADH may benefit from medication that impairs renal responsiveness to ADH. Lithium has this effect, but is usually not used because of toxicity and side effects. Demeclocycline (600–1200 mg/d) may correct serum sodium without the need for water restriction.

Anderson RJ, Chung H-M, Kluge R, et al.: Hyponatremia: a prospective analysis of its epidemiology and the pathogenetic role of vasopressin. Ann Intern Med 1985; *102*:164–168.

Beck RH, Lavizzo-Mourey R: Geriatric hyponatremia. Ann Intern Med 1987; *107*:768–769.

Cusick JF, Hagen TC, Findling JW: Inappropriate secretion of antidiuretic hormone after transsphenoidal surgery for pituitary tumors. N Engl J Med 1984; *311*:36–38.

Forrest JN, Cox M, Hong C, Morrison F, et al.: Superiority of demeclocycline over lithium in the treatment of chronic syndrome of inappropriate secretion of antidiuretic hormone. N Engl J Med 1978; *298*:173–177.

Moses AM, Notman DD: Diabetes insipidus and syndrome of inappropriate antidiuretic hormone secretion (SIADH). Adv Int Med 1982; *27*:73–100.

Rose BD: New approach to disturbances in the plasma sodium concentration. Am J Med 1986; *81*:1033–1040.

Sterns RH: Severe symptomatic hyponatremia: treatment and outcome. Ann Intern Med 1987; *107*:656–664.

Sterns RH, Riggs JE, Schochet SS Jr: Osmotic demyelination syndrome following correction of hyponatremia. N Engl J Med 1986; *314*:1535–1542.

4

Reproductive Endocrinology

Background, Pathophysiology

The normal relationships among the hypothalamus, pituitary, and mature gonads (ovaries or testes) are quite complex. A simplified scheme is shown in Figure 4–1. Gonadotropin releasing hormone (GnRH) from the hypothalamus stimulates synthesis and release of the two pituitary gonadotropins, luteinizing hormone (LH) and follicle stimulating hormone (FSH). The main effect of LH on the gonads is to regulate synthesis of sex hormones (estradiol and progesterone in females, testosterone in males); sex steroids exert feedback effects on the pituitary (negative feedback by testosterone; both negative and positive feedback by estradiol, depending on the concentration). The main effect of FSH is on gametogenesis; feedback exerted on FSH is less clear than for LH, and probably involves substances like inhibin that are produced by the gonads along with germ cells. The interplay of these hormones results in normal sexual maturation at the expected time of puberty (development of so-called secondary sex characteristics such as breast development in women, and in men, deepening of the voice and growth of hair on the face and body) and ultimately, fertility.

Hypothalamic secretion of GnRH is episodic; continuous administration of GnRH leads to suppression of gonadotropins and hypogonadism. LH, FSH, estradiol, and testosterone are also secreted episodically, following and parallelling secretion of GnRH.

Puberty. During childhood, levels of sex steroids and gonadotropins are low and similar for both sexes. The transition from sexual immaturity begins with diminished sensitivity of the pituitary or hypothalamus, or both, to negative feedback from sex steroids. LH, FSH, and gonadal steroids rise gradually to adult levels over several years. In girls, puberty typically begins between ages 8½ and 13½, first with an increase in linear growth, then the appearance of pubic hair (probably due to increased adrenal androgen secretion and termed "adren-

47

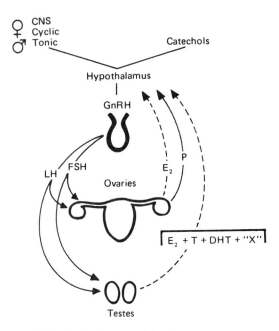

Fig. 4–1. Hypothalamic-pituitary-gonadal axis.

arche"), followed by breast development (thelarche), and finally, the onset of menses (menarche) which should occur by age 16½. In boys, puberty begins between ages 10 and 16, initially with growth in the size of the testicles, followed by deepening of the voice, enlargement of the penis, and growth of beard and body hair.

Normal Menstrual Cycle. During the normal menstrual cycle there are closely cordinated feedback effects that include the hypothalamus, the anterior pituitary gland, and the ovaries. There are also cyclic hormone changes that lead to functional and structural changes in the ovaries (follicle maturation, ovulation, and corpus luteum development), uterus (preparation of the endometrium for possible implantation of the fertilized ovum), cervix (to permit transport of sperm), and vagina. The menstrual cycle is usually counted as beginning on the first day of menstrual bleeding (day 1) and divided into three phases. The *follicular phase,* approximately the first half of the cycle (14 days of a 28-day cycle) actually begins a few days before the onset of bleeding as indicated by falling levels of estrogen and progesterone. During the early follicular phase, estrogen

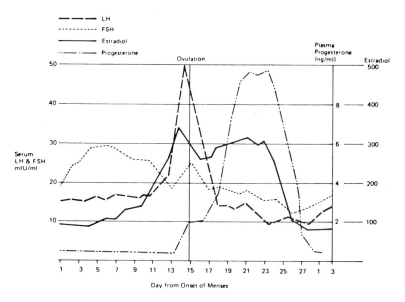

Fig. 4–2. Hormone profile of the menstrual cycle.

levels are low, causing diminished negative feedback on the pituitary-hypothalmic axis and greater secretion of LH and FSH. Progesterone secretion is also low during this phase. Toward the end of the follicular phase, estradiol rises; the higher estrogen level triggers positive feedback centers in the pituitary and hypothalamus, resulting in an increase of GnRH from the hypothalamus. This begins the *ovulatory phase,* a period of about 48 hours at midcycle when there is a rise in estradiol, LH, and FSH; this is followed by ovulation. The last half of the cycle, the *luteal phase,* is characterized by increasing production of progesterone and estrogen with gradual lowering of LH and FSH levels. A schematic presentation of the hormone changes of a normal menstrual cycle is shown in Figure 4–2. There are other hormone changes during the menstrual cycle; an androgen peak at midcycle possibly serves to increase libido at that time; estrone, an estrogen derived mainly from peripheral sources, also rises through the cycle. Estrogen and progesterone have visible effects on vaginal cytologic characteristics and cervical mucus, and progesterone elevates body temperature.

Yen SSC, Jaffe RB (eds): Reproductive Endocrinology: Physiology, Pathophysiology, and Clinical Management, 2nd ed. Philadelphia, WB Saunders, 1986.

DISORDERS OF FEMALE REPRODUCTION

Clinical Manifestations and Diagnosis

Puberty. *Precocious puberty* is more common in girls than boys. With true isosexual precocious puberty the physical and hormonal changes are identical with those of normal puberty; this may be due to central nervous system tumors or be idiopathic. Incomplete features of puberty suggest sex-hormone-producing tumors of the ovaries or adrenal glands or gonadotropin-secreting tumors. Diagnostic studies should include CT or MR of the pituitary-hypothalamic area, measurement of FSH and LH (with most assays for LH, hCG would also be measured because of structural similarities; a specific assay for hCG should be ordered if "LH" is elevated), and possibly estradiol. Appropriate imaging studies should be considered if an ovarian or adrenal tumor is suspected. *Delayed puberty* may result from chromosomal abnormalities such as Turner's syndrome or less common organic causes, but frequently is not due to disease (simply the unusually late end of the normal spectrum of maturation). If the onset of puberty is late, measurement of gonadotropins (LH and FSH) should be done; elevated levels indicate gonadal failure; chromosome analysis should be done in a girl with delayed puberty and elevated gonadotropins. If gonadotropin levels are not elevated (normal or low), further investigation may be postponed hoping for puberty to begin spontaneously, or a central defect (hypothalamus or pituitary) may be looked for with pituitary function testing and imaging. Stimulation testing with GnRH is not usually helpful in separating constitutional delayed puberty from organic causes; the response of LH and FSH to a bolus of GnRH can usually be predicted from basal values.

Hypogonadism, Ovarian Failure, and Menopause. The physical effects of gonadal steroids (or the lack of them) are easily read from evaluation of vaginal cells, cervical mucus, basal body temperature, and endometrial biopsy. Laboratory measurements of specific estrogens (such as estradiol or estrone) or total estrogens, though readily made, are relatively insensitive and rarely add much to these other clinical observations. Irregular or absent menses often indicates altered or diminished sex hormone production. (Menstrual disturbance may also result from androgen excess, prolactin excess, or systemic illness. Anatomic abnormalities that cause infertility may occur with or without endocrine abnormalities.) With advancing age, the ovaries fail to produce adequate amounts of estrogen and progesterone and ovulation ceases. Cycle length shortens and cycles become irregular, due in part to irregular maturation of the follicles, which results in anovulatory bleeding. FSH begins to rise, then fluctuates irregularly; both FSH and LH then increase as the failure of ovarian estrogen production eliminates the negative feedback effect on the pituitary. Ovarian failure may occur at any age, but prior to age 40 is considered premature, and causes other than menopause should be sought. The diagnosis of ovarian failure can be made by observing target organs for a lack of estrogen effect or demonstrating low levels of estradiol in serum or urine. Patients with ovarian failure should be investigated further to identify the site of the lesion.

Primary ovarian failure is due to abnormalities of the ovaries (such as radiation or chemotherapeutic drugs, autoimmune destruction, or resistance of the ovaries to the effects of gonadotropins) and is accompanied by a consistent elevation of plasma gonadotropin levels (LH and FSH); *secondary ovarian failure* is the result of disorders of the pituitary, hypothalamus, or higher centers, wtih deficient production of gonadotropins leading to failure of the ovaries. (The terms "primary" and "secondary," when applied to gonadal status, point to the involvement of peripheral or central glands; when applied to women with amenorrhea, "primary" means failure of menses ever to occur and "secondary" means that menses began on schedule but ceased at a later time.) Secondary ovarian failure may result from tumors or infiltrative lesions of the pituitary or hypothalamus that interfere with the production of gonadotropins or gonadotropin releasing hormone (GnRH), or from inhibition of normal gonadotropic function by excessive prolactin levels. Quite often, a specific cause for central ovarian failure cannot be found; some of the factors that have been implicated include psychologic stress and weight loss (anorexia nervosa is a striking example of both), intensive physical training, and a variety of acute and chronic diseases. It was hoped that the use of GnRH stimulation testing would elucidate the nature of the lesion in these women, but the results have been disappointing. A few cases have been reported with evidence for secretion of gonadotropins with reduced biologic activity. Hormonal measurements in these patients are the same as found in primary ovarian failure (low estrogens with elevated LH and FSH).

Amenorrhea is called "primary" when menses fail to occur spontaneously and "secondary" when menses have once begun and later stopped. *Primary amenorrhea* should be considered when menses have not begun by age 16½. The most common cause is a sex chromosome abnormality such as Turner's syndrome; these disorders are characterized by high levels of LH and FSH, low levels of estrogens, and low effects of estrogens on target tissues. *Secondary amenorrhea* is diagnosed when menses have stopped after months or years of cyclic bleeding. Causes of secondary amenorrhea are shown in Table 4–1. The extent of the evaluation should be determined by the clinical findings. Administration of progesterone for a few days will be followed by vaginal bleeding a day or two after the drug is withdrawn if the endometrium has been "primed" by estrogen, such as in polycystic ovary syndrome and some hypothalamic disorders; no bleeding will follow progesterone withdrawal if the endometrium is atrophic as a result of profound estrogen deficiency or over-aggressive curettage. LH and FSH should be measured to determine if the problem is in the ovaries (ovarian failure, with high LH and FSH) or a central one (hypothalamic or pituitary disorder, with LH and FSH "normal" or low). Prolactin determination is indicated if LH and FSH are not ele-

Table 4–1. Causes of Secondary Amenorrhea

CENTRAL
   "Higher centers"
      Anorexia nervosa
      Excessive physical training
      Psychogenic
      "Post-pill" amenorrhea
   Hypothalamic and pituitary diseases
      Hyperprolactinemia
      Destruction by neoplasm, inflammation, or vascular insult
      CNS surgery, irradiation, trauma

OVARIAN
   Polycystic ovary syndrome
   Premature ovarian failure
   Gonadotropin resistant ovary syndrome
   Gonadal dysgenesis
   Toxins, drugs, irradiation
   Oophorectomy

UTERINE
   Pregnancy, choriocarcinoma
   Asherman's syndrome (endometrial failure)

OTHER
   Systemic illness
   Thyroid and adrenal disorders

vated, particularly if galactorrhea is present. If fertility is important, a more detailed evaluation is necessary.

Infertility. In normal ovulatory menstrual cycles, bleeding usually occurs 14 or 15 days after the midcycle LH surge. Normal women display a fair amount of variation in cycle length due to differences in the length of the follicular phase. A shortened luteal phase may cause infertility; progesterone secretion is low, the corpus luteum regresses early, and menses occur only 5 to 10 days after the midcycle peak. This can be diagnosed by mid-luteal phase progesterone measurement or endometrial biopsy. In some women with infertility, cycle length may be normal but ovulation does not occur; a record of basal body temperature, profile of the pattern of gonadotropin release, or an innovative method of ovulation detection by monitoring salivary and vaginal electrical resistance (Albrecht BH, Fernando RS, Betz G: A new method for predicting and confirming ovulation. Fertil Steril 1985; *44*:200–205) may help elucidate the problem. Anatomic disorders should be looked for. Remembering that fertility requires normal male function as well as female, evaluation of infertility should include both partners.

Hirsutism. Excess growth of facial and body hair (hirsutism) is usually psychologically disturbing and may be a sign of underlying disorders. Sometimes a side effect of various medications, hirsutism may also be due to an increase in androgen production or may not have an identifiable underlying cause (idiopathic). Causes of hirsutism are shown in Table 4–2. Evaluation should begin with a complete history regarding drugs and other affected family members, and physical examination

Table 4–2. Causes of Hirsutism

Medications
    Minoxidil, diazoxide, phenytoin, glucocorticoids, cyclosporin, androgens, anabolic steroids
Endocrine disorders
    Adrenal disorders
        Congenital adrenal hyperplasia (classic and "late-onset")
        Androgen-secreting tumors
        ACTH-dependent Cushing's syndrome
    Ovarian disorders
        Polycystic ovary syndrome
        Hyperthecosis, hilus-cell or stromal cell hyperplasia
        Androgen-secreting tumors
        Insulin resistance-androgen excess
    Combined adrenal-ovarian androgen excess (nonspecific)
    Familial
    Idiopathic

for evidence of virilism (clitoral enlargement, deepening of the voice, male pattern baldness) which would suggest an androgen-producing tumor. Signs of androgen excess associated with signs of glucocorticoid excess such as central obesity, hypertension, etc., would suggest Cushing's syndrome and should be evaluated with urinary free cortisol or an overnight dexamethasone suppression test (see Cushing's syndrome, p. 99). There are a variety of nontumorous causes of androgen excess; the excess androgen may come from the adrenal glands, the ovaries, peripheral conversion of steroid precursors to androgens by skin and other tissues, or a combination of these. Only a few women with hirsutism have an identifiable underlying disorder (such as congenital adrenal hyperplasia; see chapter on the adrenal glands).

While there are a number of androgenic hormones, measurement of two of these provides the basic information needed to evaluate a patient with hirsutism. Dehydroepiandrosterone sulfate (DHEAS) is a relatively weak androgen derived almost exclusively from the adrenal glands and is usually elevated when adrenal androgen excess is present. Testosterone is derived from the ovaries, adrenals, and peripheral precursors. Plasma DHEAS ≥ 700 µg/dL is strongly suggestive of an adrenal tumor that is secreting androgens. Total serum testosterone ≥ 200 ng/dL suggests a testosterone-producing tumor; these tumors are usually found in the ovaries but may also arise in the adrenal glands. If enough different androgens are measured (such as free testostosterone rather than total, androstenedione, etc.), "abnormalities" are found in most hirsute women. However, simply finding an elevation of one of these compounds does not provide a definitive diagnosis; no matter how precise or controlled the measurement in an individual patient, determination of basal androgen levels in blood or urine may suggest but does not conclusively identify the source of the androgen production. An elevated level of DHEAS with a normal total testosterone value points to an adrenal origin for androgen excess, whereas elevated total testosterone but normal DHEAS indicates ovarian androgen excess. Elevation of both DHEAS and total testosterone indicates a mixed source of the androgens. Treatment can be based on these two measurements, with the patient categorized as idiopathic hirsutism, adrenal androgen excess, ovarian androgen excess, or mixed.

Androgen production at the hair follicle itself may be an additional factor in hirsutism. Testosterone is converted to a more active form, dihydrotestosterone, by the enzyme 5-alpha reductase in the skin; 3-alpha-androstanediol glucuronide is a metabolically inert end-product of degradation of dihydrotestosterone in target tissues; its measurement seems promising as a means to identify women with hirsutism due to increased end-organ sensitivity, and may reduce the number of women diagnosed as having "idiopathic" hirsutism.

Treatment

Treatment of *precocious puberty* has advanced considerably with the availability of gonadotropin releasing hormone antagonists (Naferelin) and agonists of GnRH, which inhibit release of gonadotropins when administered continuously. Agents such as progesterone and danazole are helpful but not completely satisfactory. *Delayed puberty* in females may be managed with watchful waiting, or, if acceleration of secondary sexual characteristics is desired, by administration of estrogens. If the problem lies in the hypothalamus, GnRH administered in pulses by an infusion pump may be considered.

Therapy of *ovarian failure* depends in part on the specific goals and desires of the patient. In women with primary ovarian disease, fertility can be achieved only rarely (though occasional success has been reported with glucocorticoids in autoimmune ovarian failure or high-dose gonadotropin or estrogen treatment in the rare condition called the gonadotropin-resistant ovary syndrome). However, if the problem is in the pituitary, hypothalamus, or higher centers, ovulation and conception are realistic aims. With pituitary or hypothalamic failure, ovulation can be induced using a combination of human menopausal gonadotropins (Pergonal) and human chorionic gonadotropin (A.P.L., Glukor, Profasi). This therapy is associated with an increased frequency of multiple births and can cause severe ovarian hyperstimulation; it should be limited to specialized centers with proven expertise. As mentioned in regard to delayed puberty, recent studies suggest that women with hypothalamic disease can achieve ovulation with pulsatile administration of gonadotropin-releasing hormone (GnRH). In women with hyperprolactinemia, bromocriptine (Parlodel) usually restores normal reproductive function.

If estrogen deficiency occurs, replacement therapy should be continued at least until the expected age of the menopause (age 50) and perhaps longer, to minimize the rapid loss of bone that occurs in the hypoestrogenemic state. Most of the troublesome signs and symptoms of ovarian failure (hot flashes and vaginal dryness) are relieved by estrogen treatment. Estrogen-deficient

55

women are at increased risk for coronary heart disease and osteoporosis; in the absence of specific contraindications, continuing estrogen treatment lifelong may be appropriate.

It is advisable to give estrogen cyclically in combination with progesterone to avoid endometrial hyperplasia or endometrial carcinoma. A typical schedule is conjugated or esterified estrogens (Estratab, Menrium, Premarin) 0.625 or 1.25 mg orally in days 1 through 25 monthly and medroxyprogesterone acetate (Amen, Curretab, Provera) 10 mg orally on days 11 through 25 monthly. In some women, conjugated estrogens are not fully satisfactory in relieving symptoms; oral micronized estradiol (Estrace) in a dose of 1 or 2 mg daily may be substituted for conjugated estrogens and is often effective. Intravaginal estrogen creams relieve vaginal dryness but are sufficiently absorbed to provide a systemic effect, and so should be given cyclically with progesterone. Transdermal preparations of estradiol are now available (Estraderm) and show some promise, though skin irritation has been a problem. Orally administered estrogens pass through the liver and influence the synthesis of a variety of proteins that may be beneficial (such as HDL cholesterol), of no clinical consequence (such as thyroxine binding globulin) or potentially detrimental (antithrombin III, fibrinogen, renin substrate). These hepatic effects are not seen with transdermal estradiol; whether this is due to the route of administration or just differences between estradiol and conjugated estrogens is not yet clear. Estrogens can be given continuously and without progesterone in women who have had a hysterectomy.

Estrogens are contraindicated in women with estrogen-dependent tumors such as carcinoma of the breast. Cycling estrogen with progesterone eliminates the risk of endometrial carcinoma seen with continuous, unopposed estrogen. Menstrual bleeding is likely to continue when estrogen treatment is given, and this may be a significant drawback to continuing treatment after the expected age of menopause; preliminary studies suggest that combining a small daily dose of a progestational agent with daily estrogen will result in endometrial atrophy which would eliminate this drawback. Some women taking estrogens develop troublesome breast tenderness or worsening of fibrocystic breast disease. Estrogen treatment is associated with an increased risk of gallstones, and, in some women, may cause or aggravate thromboembolic disorders, systemic arterial hypertension, edema, or glucose intolerance.

Management of *amenorrhea* and *infertility* must be individualized based on the specific diagnosis and pathophysiology.

Hirsutism can be managed with cosmetic measures such as bleaching, wax depilatories, plucking, shaving, or electrolysis. However, if there is a significant hormone abnormality, medical treatment should be added to minimize the growth of new hair. Mild adrenal androgen excess not due to neoplasm usually can be corrected with a low dose of glucocorticoid (prednisone 5 mg given at bedtime to blunt the night-time ACTH surge), and ovarian androgen excess corrected with cyclic estrogen and progesterone (either given as individual agents or as birth control pills). Spironolactone 100 to 200 mg daily may cause some regression of hair growth, probably from direct effects on the hair follicle. Patients should be counselled that with medical treatment existing hair will regress little and slowly, if at all.

Board JA, Rosenberg SM, Smeltzer JS: Spironolactone and estrogen-progestin therapy for hirsutism. South Med J 1987; *80*:483–486.

Bullen BA, Skrinar GS, Beitins IZ, et al.: Induction of menstrual disorders by strenuous exercise in untrained women. N Engl J Med 1985; *312*:1349–1353.

Chetkowski RJ, Meldrum DR, Steingold KA, et al.: Biologic effects of transdermal estradiol. N Engl J Med 1986; *314*:1615–1620.

Coulam CB: Premature gonadal failure. Fertil Steril 1982; *38*:645–655.

(Council on Scientific Affairs) Estrogen replacement in the menopause. JAMA 1983; *249*:359–361.

Cutler GB (moderator): Therapeutic applications of luteinizing-hormone-releasing hormone and its analogs. Ann Intern Med 1985; *102*:643–657.

Magos AL, Brincat M, Studd JWW, et al.: Amenorrhea and endometrial atrophy with continuous oral estrogen and progestogen therapy in postmenopausal women. Obstet Gynecol 1985; *65*:496–499.

Marshall JC, Kelch RP: Gonadotropin-releasing hormone: role of pulsatile secretion in the regulation of reproduction. N Engl J Med 1986; *315*:1459–1468.

McKenna TJ: Pathogenesis and treatment of polycystic ovary syndrome. N Engl J Med 1988; *318*:558–562.

Moghissi KS, Wallach EE: Unexplained infertility. Fertil Steril 1983; *39*:5–21.

Ravnikar V, Elking-Hirsch K, Shiff I, et al.: Vasomotor flushes and the release of peripheral immunoreactive luteinizing hormone-releasing hormone. Fertil Steril 1984; *41*:881–884.

Reid RL, Van Vugt DA: Weight-related changes in reproductive function. Fertil Steril 1987; *48*:905–913.

Rittmaster RS, Loriau DL: Hirsutism. Ann Intern Med 1987; *106*:95–107.

Root AW, Shulman DI: Isosexual precocity: current concepts and recent advances. Fertil Steril 1986; *45*:749–766.

Schlaff WD: Dynamic testing in reproductive endocrinolgoy. Fertil Steril 1986; *45*:589–606.

Vermesh M, Kletzky OA, Davajan V, et al.: Monitoring techniques to predict and detect ovulation. Fertil Steril 1987; *47*:259–265.

Wentz AC, Herbert CM III, Hill GA: Gynecologic Endocrinology and Infertility for the House Officer. Baltimore, Williams and Wilkins, 1988.

DISORDERS OF MALE REPRODUCTION

Clinical Manifestations and Diagnosis

Puberty. *Precocious puberty* in males is usually due to a central nervous system lesion or is idiopathic. *Delayed puberty* is often simply the late end of the normal spectrum of development but may be due to congenital or acquired abnormalities of the testes, pituitary, or hypothalamus (Table 4–3). The site of the defect may be determined using hormone measurements as outlined under hypogonadism.

Male Hypogonadism, Impotence, and Infertility. If the onset of hypogonadism is before puberty, male secondary sex characteristics fail to develop and growth of the long bones continues past the usual time of epiphyseal closure, resulting in "eunuchoid" habitus where the ratio of upper to lower body segment is less than 1 and arm span is greater than height. Acquired hypogonadism, presenting after puberty, is manifest by diminished libido, impotence, and infertility; if hypogonadism is severe and prolonged, beard growth may diminish. Generally, the cause of male hypogonadism can be classified by using hormone measurements. A simplified classification includes (1) deficient secretion of LH and FSH due to abnor-

Table 4–3. Causes of Delayed Puberty in Males

Hypogonadotropic
    Kallman's syndrome (hypogonadotropic hypogonadism)
    Isolated LH deficiency
    Craniopharyngioma, pituitary, other CNS tumor
    Inflammation, radiation, vascular insult, trauma
    Prader-Willi syndrome
    Lawrence-Moon-Biedl syndrome

Hypergonadotropic
    Congenital anorchia
    Androgen resistance syndromes
    Chromosomal abnormalities (e.g., Klinefelter's syndrome)
    Noonan syndrome ("male Turner's")

Other
    Systemic illness, malnutrition
    Thyroid and adrenal disorders
    Constitutional delay of growth

malities in hypothalamic or pituitary function (secondary hypogonadism); (2) primary gonadal abnormalities; and (3) defective end organ responsiveness due to chemical or cellular defects in androgen synthesis, androgen action, or both. Measurement of serum testosterone, LH, and FSH provides the necessary initial data. In primary hypogonadism, LH and FSH are elevated but testosterone is low. When hypogonadism is secondary to pituitary or hypothalamic hypofunction, LH, FSH, and testosterone are all low. Less commonly, germ cell failure will be found, with elevated FSH but normal LH and testosterone. In syndromes of partial androgen resistance, LH is increased, FSH is normal, and testosterone is normal or increased.

The pituitary-gonadal axis may be affected by a number of systemic diseases. Chronic renal failure causes a decrease in testosterone and sperm count, but LH and FSH levels are not elevated. With chronic cirrhosis, testosterone concentration tends to be low and estrogen levels elevated, but plasma LH and FSH are in the normal range. Even in the absence of liver disease, alcohol may have a direct effect on the testes, impairing spermatogenesis. With severe malnutrition, plasma testosterone declines but LH is variably affected (normal or low). Cortisol excess and deficiency states, thyroid hormone excess and deficiency states, or any chronic debilitating illness may affect reproductive hormone levels and sexual function.

Impotence is the persistent inability to develop or maintain a penile erection sufficient for intercourse and ejaculation. Impotence may result from psychogenic causes, a variety of medications, vascular insufficiency, and neuropathy, in addition to hypogonadism. Evaluation should include a complete history and physical examination. If there is no obvious explanation for troublesome impotence, LH and FSH measurements are indicated; elevated values establish a diagnosis of primary hypogonadism. Total and even free testosterone levels may be in the normal range for adult males yet may still be subnormal for a specific individual, as indicated by elevated LH or FSH values. Hyperprolactinemia is an infrequent cause of impotence but should be considered in unusual situations.

Male infertility may be due to a variety of causes as shown in Table 4–4. The investigation of *infertility* in males should begin with semen analysis. Infertility is rarely the sole presentation of primary or secondary hypogonadism in men; other clinical features, particularly impotence, generally point to that diagnosis. A low sperm count may result from anatomic abnormalities, including varicocele. Hyperprolactinemia may

59

Table 4–4. Causes of Male Infertility

Irreversible	Potentially Reversible
Chromosome abnormalities	Vas or epididymal occlusion
Absent vas deferens	Retrograde ejaculation
Nonmotile sperm	Prostatitis, epididymitis
Mumps orchitis	Varicocele
Cryptorchidism	Gonadotropin or GnRH
Toxins	deficiency
Epididymal dysfunction	Drugs
	Heat
	Immunologic
	Systemic illness
	Sexual dysfunction

cause oligospermia as well as secondary hypogonadism. Unless evidence of androgen deficiency is present, endocrine profiles in patients with oligospermia generally are not helpful.

Gynecomastia. The presence of glandular breast tissue in pubertal males is common and almost always resolves spontaneously. In adult males, the growth of glandular breast tissue should be viewed with suspicion. Gynecomastia may be unilateral or bilateral; unilateral gynecomastia has no specific diagnostic significance. Gynecomastia may develop due to excessive use of alcohol, marijuana, or certain medications, or may be associated with hyperthyroidism or hypothyroidism. Chromosomal abnormalities such as Klinefelter's syndrome are often accompanied by gynecomastia, but hypogonadism is usually obvious in these patients. Germinal-cell or nonendocrine tumors that produce chorionic gonadotropin; estrogen-producing tumors of the adrenals, testes, or liver; and prolactin-producing pituitary adenomas all may cause gynecomastia. These are uncommon disorders, and the cause of gynecomastia will remain unknown in many cases. When history and physical examination do not point to a specific disorder, measurement of hCG, plasma estradiol (or total estrogens), and prolactin are appropriate.

Treatment

Precocious puberty is best managed by suppressing gonadotropin secretion with an agonist or antagonist of GnRH. Sexual maturation in males with *delayed puberty* can be hastened without long-term adverse effects on reproductive function by injections of testosterone; or by administration of chorionic gonadotropin (hCG), which, like LH, stimulates testosterone synthesis; or by pulsatile administration of GnRH.

Treatment of *hypogonadism* depends on the cause and the patient's goals. Testosterone replacement is indicated for primary hypogonadism and for secondary hypogonadism if immediate fertility is not desired. This can be provided using a long-acting injectable form of testosterone (testosterone enanthate or cipionate, 200 mg IM every 2 weeks). When fertility is desired, hypogonadism due to pituitary or hypothalamic disease may be treated by co-administration of hCG to stimulate testosterone production and FSH (human menopausal gonadotropins, hMG) to stimulate gametogenesis. Patients with hypothalamic disorders may respond to pulsatile administration of GnRH.

Treatment of *impotence* and *infertility* depends on the specific cause and goals of the patient. *Gynecomastia* does not respond well to medical treatment; tenderness may be treated symptomatically (analgesics, warm soaks) but surgery may be needed to reduce breast size and relieve psychologic distress.

Carlson HE: Gynecomastia. N Engl J Med 1980; *303*:795–800.

Morley JE: Impotence. Am J Med 1986; *80*:897–905.

Swerdloff RS, Boyers SP: Evaluation of the male partner of an infertile couple: An algorithmic approach. JAMA 1982; *247*:2418–2422.

Swerdloff RS (moderator): Infertility in the male. Ann Intern Med 1985; *103*:906–919.

$$\overline{5}$$

Thyroid Gland

Background, Pathophysiology

The thyroid gland lies in the anterior neck, two lobes connected by a thin band of tissue, the isthmus, giving the gland the configuration of a butterfly. Thyroid follicles consist of a layer of epithelial cells enclosing amorphous material called colloid, composed of an iodinated glycoprotein, thyroglobulin. The thyroid also contains parafollicular cells (C cells) which produce the hormone calcitonin.

Iodine transport into the follicles is the first and rate-limiting step in thyroid hormone synthesis. After oxidation to iodide it is bound to tyrosine molecules that are attached to thyroglobulin in the colloid. Monoiodotyrosine (MIT) and diiodotyrosine (DIT) are formed; two DIT molecules condense to form T_4, still linked to thyroglobulin. Similarly, T_3 and a small amount of rT_3 result from combination of MIT and DIT.

Thyroxine (T_4) is the primary secretory product of the thyroid gland, which also produces smaller amounts of triiodothyronine (T_3). In peripheral tissues, particularly the liver, T_4 undergoes deiodination of the outer ring at the 5' position to yield T_3 (which is 4 to 5 times more potent metabolically than T_4). At least 80% of T_3 and essentially all reverse T_3 (rT_3, an inactive compound produced by removal of an iodine from the inner ring of T_4) result from deiodination of T_4 by the liver and other peripheral tissues rather than from direct secretion from the thyroid. Figure 5–1 shows the structure and relative potency of the important products of the thyroid gland. Deiodination of T_4 is a rapidly responsive mechanism for control of thyroid hormone balance; acute or chronic stress or illness causes a shift in the direction of this deiodination, favoring formation of the inactive product, reverse T_3, rather than the more active T_3, though the T_4 level remains essentially unchanged. Various medications also shift peripheral deiodination toward inactive rT_3 (Table 5–1).

In the circulation T_4 and T_3 are reversibly bound to carrier proteins (thyroxine-binding globulin, thyroxine-binding preal-

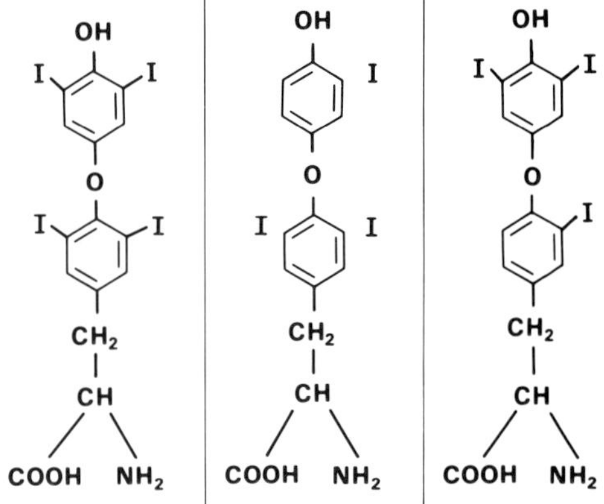

Fig. 5–1. Structure, potency, and derivation of thyroid hormones.

	T_4	T_3	rT_3
Potency (relative to T_4)	1	4+	0
Percent derived from thyroidal secretion	100%	<20%	<10%
Percent derived from peripheral conversion	0	>80%	>90%

Table 5–1. Factors that Inhibit Peripheral Conversion of T_4 to T_3

Fasting, malnutrition
Acute and chronic nonthyroidal illness
Drugs:
    Propranolol
    Glucocorticoids
    Iodinated contrast agents (e.g., ipodate)
    Propylthiouracil
    Amiodarone

bumin, and albumin) which bind 99.97% of T_4 and 99.7% of T_3; only the small free fraction of each hormone is biologically active. Because of the large variation in the concentration of thyroxine-binding proteins under normal circumstances, there is wide variation in total T_4 levels among euthyroid individuals. Total T_3 concentrations also vary with alterations in the concentrations of binding proteins, although not as much as T_4. Common circumstances in which thyroid hormone-binding proteins are altered are shown in Table 5–2. When using thyroid hormone measurements to diagnose thyroid hormone excess or deficiency states, knowledge of possible changes in the concentration of binding proteins or free hormone is extremely important.

Although thyroid hormones have many actions, the primary one is to increase energy expenditure (oxygen consumption) in many tissues. Thyroid hormones are required for growth, development, and sexual maturation. Other actions include stimulation of cardiac contraction, maintenance of body weight, stimulation of protein synthesis and carbohydrate metabolism, increase in the synthesis and degradation of cholesterol and triglycerides, increase in vitamin requirements, and enhancement of sensitivity of the beta-adrenergic receptors to catecholamines.

Thyrotropin-releasing hormone (TRH), a tripeptide produced in the hypothalamus, acts on the pituitary to cause the synthesis and release of thyroid-stimulating hormone (TSH). TSH in turn controls synthesis and release of thyroid hormones as well as inducing an increase in the size and number of thyroidal follicular cells. A rise in thyroid hormone level inhibits the pituitary response to TRH (negative feedback); a fall in thyroid hormones causes an increase in TRH and TSH secretion (Fig. 5–2).

Common disorders of the thyroid include (1) thyroid hormone excess or deficiency (hyper- and hypothyroidism), (2) diffuse or nodular thyroid enlargement (goiter), and (3) thyroiditis. Often, there is overlap between these categories (e.g., goitrous hypothyroidism, or hyperthyroidism due to diffuse toxic goiter with coexistent chronic lymphocytic thyroiditis).

Laboratory Diagnosis of Thyroid Dysfunction

Clinical signs and symptoms of thyroid hormone excess and deficiency are nonspecific. Laboratory tests are usually relied

Table 5–2. Factors Associated with Changes in Serum Thyroid Hormone Binding Proteins

Increase	Decrease
Drugs: estrogens, perphenazine, clofibrate, heroin, morphine	Drugs: androgens, danazol, anabolic steroids, glucocorticoids
Pregnancy	Major illness or stress
Acute intermittent porphyria	Nephrotic syndrome
Infectious hepatitis	Active acromegaly
Genetically determined	Genetically determined

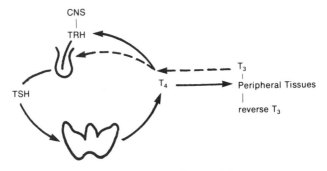

Fig. 5–2. Hypothalamic-pituitary-thyroid feedback loop.

Table 5–3. Commonly Used Thyroid Tests

T_4	Thyroxine; total serum T_4
FT_4	Free T_4 by dialysis (or other method)
FT_4I	Free T_4 index (calculated, $T_4 \times T_3RU$); estimate of free T_4
T_3	Triiodothyronine; total serum T_3; also called T_3 (RIA)
T_3RU	T_3 resin uptake, an assessment of binding protein; does not reflect T_3 levels in vivo; recently suggested nomenclature is THBR (thyroid hormone binding ratio)
rT_3	Reverse T_3; metabolically inactive
TBG	Thyroxine binding globulin
TSH	Thyroid stimulating hormone
TRH	Thyrotropin-releasing hormone; not usually measured directly, but used to stimulate TSH
RaIU	Radioactive iodine uptake; percent of administered dose taken up by the thyroid in specified time (usually 24 h)

on for diagnosis of hyper-or hypothyroidism; the most commonly used tests are listed in Table 5–3. Normal thyroid hormone levels do not exclude thyroid disease, abnormal thyroid tests do not always indicate thyroid disease, and diffuse or nodular thyroid enlargement may be seen in euthyroid patients.

Conventionally, thyroid testing has been done stepwise, with the initial step being one of three methods: (1) a total thyroxine measurement, (2) calculation of free thyroxine index (FTI) from total T_4 and T_3 uptake ratio measurements, or (3) one of the newer analog assays for free thyroxine (FT_4) measurement. Total T_4 is a good reflection of thyroid hormone production. However, changes in serum thyroid hormone binding proteins affect total T_4 levels without changing the free, active hormone ("abnormal" tests in the absence of thyroid disease). Most changes in binding protein can be corrected for with the FTI or FT_4 (though extreme binding protein variations often give abnormal FTI or FT_4 results). For initial testing, total T_4, T_3 uptake, and calculated FTI provide more reliable information than a total T_4 value alone and more useful information than the single test, FT_4.

T_4, FTI, and FT_4 are not ideal indicators of thyroid status, not only because of binding protein variations, but also because T_3 is the primary active thyroid hormone and the relationships between these hormones (T_4 and T_3) are not always predictable. This will be discussed later in more detail. In hyperthyroidism, T_3 is typically elevated to a greater degree than T_4. Because T_3 levels fluctuate rapidly in response to stress and other nonthyroidal factors and are low not only in hypothyroidism but also in many other conditions, measurement of T_3 is not the ideal test of thyroid function status.

A good way to assess thyroid function is to determine the effect of thyroid hormone in one of its target tissues. While there is not yet a perfect test, the level of TSH does indicate the action of thyroid hormone in one of its target tissues: the pituitary cells that secrete TSH. Clinical use of TSH measurement has been limited by the lack of assay sensitivity—the inability of most assays to differentiate the lower limit of normal from the abnormally low. Improvements in assay technique have led to the increasing availability of TSH assays with sufficient sensitivity to distinguish low levels from normal. This is beginning to revolutionize thyroid function testing; instead of starting with a measurement of thyroid hormones—T_4, FTI, FT_4, T_3—a sensitive TSH assay is becoming accepted as the initial test of thyroid function: high in hypothyroidism, and low in hyperthyroidism or pituitary-hypothalamic disease; results that are equivocal or do not fit the clinical picture should be followed up with other tests (Fig. 5–3). TSH measurement is more reliable in the diagnosis of thyroid hormone abnormalities than thyroid hormone levels. Often, patients have normal levels of T_4 or T_3 or both, no overt clinical signs or symptoms of thyroid dysfunction, but TSH is abnormally high or low. Not all such "subclinical" thyroid disease warrants treatment, but detection of even mild thyroid function changes is important in specific patients.

Thyroid Scan, Uptake, and Ultrasound

Radioisotopes of iodine and technetium are taken up by the thyroid gland and can be used to provide an image of functioning thyroid tissue. *Scans* are useful in determining the etiology of hyperthyroidism (diffuse hyperfunction in Graves' disease, heterogeneous function in toxic multinodular goiter).

67

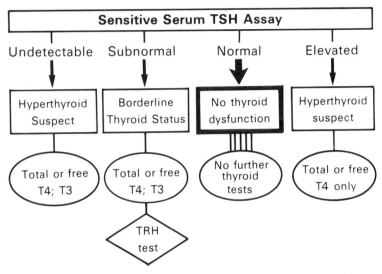

Fig. 5-3. Diagnosis of thyroid dysfunction. From Klee GG, Hay ID, Scheme for diagnosis of thyroid dysfunction. J Clin Endocrinol Metab 64:461–466, copyright by The Endocrine Society, 1987.

Thyroid scans are often used to evaluate thyroid nodules but provide such limited information that they should not be used routinely. If a thyroid scan is to be done, the isotope used for scanning is important. I-123 is the isotope of choice for studying thyroid nodules, but availability of this isotope is limited; I-131 gives equivalent results but exposes the patient to more irradiation. Technetium-99 has less radiation exposure and a 20 to 30-minute completion time (radioactive iodine scans are generally begun one day and completed 24 hours later). In many centers, Tc-99 is routinely used. However, some nodules that are "hot" on technetium scan are "cold" on iodine scan, and it is the demonstration of function on iodine scan that is significant. Finally, not all palpable abnormalities can be seen on scan; in one series, over 30% of patients with palpable thyroid carcinomas had a normal scan!

Often thought of together as "thyroid scan and uptake," these are actually two separate procedures. Quantitating the amount of isotope taken up and retained by the gland provides another parameter of thyroid function. The *thyroidal uptake of iodine* depends in part on body iodine stores, and so is lowered by high dietary iodine or exposure to exogenous iodine in medications or x-ray contrast dyes. Although radioactive iodine uptake is elevated in most forms of hyperthyroidism, it is also elevated in iodine deficiency and in some stages of Hashimoto's thyroiditis (when thyroid hormone levels are normal or low). Iodine uptake is low in some forms of hyperthyroidism (subacute or painless thyrotoxic thyroiditis, thyrotoxicosis factitia). The results must be interpreted in clinical context. Radioiodine uptake is rarely useful in the evaluation of hypothyroid patients.

Thyroid ultrasonography provides an objective measurement of thyroid anatomy (goiter, nodules); current high resolution equipment is able to detect nodules as small as 2 mm in diameter. Careful physical examination by an experienced clinician, while not able to detect such small abnormalities, provides adequate information in most patients, with ultrasound being reserved for patients where physical findings are equivocal. Thyroid ultrasound is 90 to 95% accurate in determining whether a nodule is solid, cystic, or mixed; if needle aspiration of the nodule is to be done, this determination can be made with greater accuracy and with less expense than ultrasound. Routine ultrasound of thyroid nodules is not recommended.

DeGroot JL, Larsen PR, Refetoff S, et al.: (eds): The Thyroid And Its Diseases, 5th Ed. New York, Wiley Medical, 1985.

Ingbar SH, Braverman LE (eds): Werner's The Thyroid, 5th Ed. Philadelphia, JB Lippincott, 1986.

Jackson IMD: Thyrotropin-releasing hormone. N Engl J Med 1982; *306*:145–155.

Larsen PR: Thyroid-pituitary interaction. N Engl J Med 1982; *306*:23–31.

Schimmel M, Utiger RD: Thyroidal and peripheral production of thyroid hormones: review of recent finding and their clinical implications. Ann Intern Med 1977; *87*:760–768.

HYPOTHYROIDISM

Background, Pathophysiology

Primary hypothyroidism is a common disorder, affecting 1 to 2% of the population. Primary hypothyroidism results when the thyroid gland is damaged, such as in chronic lymphocytic thyroiditis; or from inherited conditions where thyroid hormone synthesis is inefficient, such as enzyme abnormalities associated with dyshormonogenesis; or after ablation or removal of thyroid tissue with radioactive iodine or surgery. Goiter (thyroid enlargement) may be present or not, depending on the underlying cause.

Congenital hypothyroidism may be due to absence of the

thyroid gland (athyreosis) or to defects of thyroid hormone synthesis. This disorder occurs once in every 3500 to 4000 live births. Early diagnosis and treatment are critical in preventing mental retardation. Screening programs for congenital hypothyroidism have been established in most states.

Secondary hypothyroidism occurs from pituitary or hypothalamic disorders that produce a deficiency of either TRH or TSH or both. TSH deficiency rarely occurs as an isolated entity. Most patients with secondary hypothyroidism have other pituitary hormone deficiencies as well.

Clinical Presentation

Signs and symptoms of thyroid hormone deficiency include weight gain, lethargy, coarse and dry skin, constipation, cold intolerance, delayed relaxation of deep tendon reflexes, and deepening and hoarseness of the voice (Table 5–4). These symptoms are nonspecific, and not uncommonly occur in the absence of thyroid dysfunction. In early or mild hypothyroidism symptoms are often subtle, so a high degree of clinical suspicion is needed to order the appropriate tests and establish or rule out the diagnosis. On physical examination, special attention should be paid to palpation of the thyroid (enlargement or atrophy would support a diagnosis of hypothyroidism) and the relaxation speed of the Achilles reflexes.

Diagnosis of Hypothyroidism

Except in longstanding or severe hypothyroidism, the diagnosis is based on an elevated TSH level, not clinical grounds. The decrease in circulating levels of thyroid hormones leads to an increase in TSH, which can be measured to confirm a diagnosis of primary hypothyroidism. Thyroid hormone levels (T_4 or FT_4) are only slightly more reliable than clinical judgment in diagnosing hypothyroidism; in mild or early thyroid failure,

Table 5–4. Symptoms and Signs of Hypothyroidism

Symptoms	Signs
Weight gain	Growth retardation
Easy fatigue	Deep, hoarse voice
Lethargy	Dry, coarse skin
Cold intolerance	Myxedema
Hair loss	High cholesterol
Constipation	Bradycardia
	Hypertension
	Slow reflex relaxation

thyroid hormone levels may still be above the lower limit of the reference range, but TSH will be elevated. The etiology of primary hypothyroidism may be apparent by history (previous history of ablative treatment, family history of heritable defects in thyroid hormone synthesis) or suspected from physical examination (the firm, pebbly goiter of Hashimoto's thyroiditis). Although establishing the etiology of hypothyroidism is often not of clinical importance, other studies such as antimicrosomal antibodies or thyroidal uptake with perchlorate discharge may be of use in selected patients.

In secondary hypothyroidism, serum thyroid hormone concentrations are low but TSH is either within the normal range (inappropriately low for the low T_4) or only slightly elevated. When T_4 and TSH are both low and secondary hypothyroidism is suspected, the TRH stimulation test (protocol, p. 218) may be used to establish the diagnosis or to distinguish hypothalamic from pituitary disease (though this distinction is not usually important). In patients with pituitary lesions, no response of TSH to TRH is expected; with hypothalamic abnormalities, the peak TSH response to TRH may be normal but is generally delayed until 45 or 60 minutes after TRH administration rather than the usual time of 20 to 30 minutes.

Treatment of Hypothyroidism

Treatment of hypothyroidism, whether primary or secondary, is quite satisfactory. L-thyroxine can be given orally (or intravenously); the half-life is about 8 days. An average dose of L-thyroxine can be calculated by multiplying the patient's body weight in pounds by 0.75 µg per day (e.g., 100 pounds × 0.75 µg equals a dose of 75 µg/day); elderly patients may require a lower dose. For healthy, young patients with mild or moderate hypothyroidism, a full replacement dose may be started. For elderly patients or patients with underlying medical problems such as heart disease, treatment should be started with a small dose and increased gradually to full replacement. Since most circulating T_3 is derived from T_4, athyreotic patients on appropriate doses of L-thyroxine have normal circulating levels of T_3. Thyroid hormone preparations containing both T_4 and T_3 (e.g., desiccated thyroid, thyroglobulin tablets, liotrix) should not be used for routine replacement, because the exogenous T_3 often results in excessive serum T_3 levels, even when serum T_4 is normal. Once hypothyroidism has developed, lifelong treatment and followup are usually necessary.

Treatment should be monitored regularly with TSH and T_4

71

measurements and adjusted until TSH is in the normal range with T_4 or FT_4 levels that are normal or minimally elevated. Initial tests should be done after the patient has been receiving a stable dose for 6 to 8 weeks, then repeated yearly or at any time signs or symptoms of thyroid hormone excess or deficiency are present.

Myxedema Coma

Myxedema coma is a serious complication of long standing and severe hypothyroidism, often precipitated by identifiable factors such as infection, analgesics, or sedative/tranquilizers. In addition to the expected manifestations of hypothyroidism (such as delayed reflexes, or thick, cool, dry skin), patients with myxedema coma have hypoventilation, hypothermia, hypotension, and bradycardia. The goal of thyroid hormone treatment in myxedema coma is to restore normal free hormone levels as rapidly as possible; there is disagreement regarding the best preparation, dose, and route for thyroid hormone replacement. Most authorities use intravenous L-thyroxine, loading dose of 500 μg and daily maintenance dose of 100 μg. T_3, 25 μg every 6 hours (IV or orally) has been recommended. While T_3 treatment has some theoretical advantages over T_4, there are no data to indicate any real difference between these approaches. Since intravenous T_4 is available and intravenous T_3 must be prepared locally, treatment could be started with IV T_4, and T_3 added when oral or nasogastric administration is possible.

Adjunctive treatment for myxedema coma should include identification and treatment of any precipitating factors (empiric coverage with antibiotics if no factors are apparent), careful warming to restore normal core temperature, and volume expansion with pressor agents as needed to maintain perfusion. Mechanical ventilation may be needed. Stress doses of glucocorticoids (e.g., hydrocortisone 100 mg IV q 8 h) are usually given, reasoning that steroid synthesis may be slowed in hypothyroidism, or that previously undiagnosed adrenal insufficiency is present. Even with the best treatment, mortality of myxedema coma approaches 50% of cases.

Brennan MD: Thyroid hormones. Mayo Clin Proc 1980; 55:33–44.
Cooper DS: Subclinical hypothyroidism. JAMA 1987; 258:246–247.
Cooper DS, Halpern R, Wood LC, et al.: L-thyroxine therapy in subclinical hypothyroidism: A double-blind, placebo-controlled trial. Ann Intern Med 1984; 101:18–24.
(Editorial): Outcome of screening for congenital hypothyroidism. Lancet 1986; 1:1130–1129.

Fish LH, Schwartz HL, Cavanaugh J, et al.: Replacement dose, metabolism, and bioavailability of levothyroxine in the treatment of hypothyroidism: Role of triiodothyronine in pituitary feedback in humans. N Engl J Med 1987; *316*:764–770.

Hershman JM: Important role of serum TSH in the diagnosis of hypothyroidism. Thyroid Clinics 1981; *1*:1–6.

Jackson IMD, Cobb WE: Why does anyone still use desiccated thyroid USP? Am J Med 1978; *64*:284–288.

Klein I, Levey GS: Unusual manifestations of hypothyroidism. Arch Intern Med 1984; *144*:123–128.

Nicoloff JT: Thyroid storm and myxedema coma. Med Clin North Am 1985; *69*:1005–1017.

Robuschi G, Safran M, Braverman LE, et al.: Hypothyroidism in the elderly. Endocrine Reviews 1987; *8*:142–153.

Watts NB: Use of sensitive thyrotropin assay for monitoring treatment with L-thyroxine. Arch Intern Med, in press.

HYPERTHYROIDISM

Background, Pathophysiology

Hyperthyroidism can be caused by a number of conditions (Table 5–5). The most common form, diffuse toxic goiter (Graves' disease) results from the presence of autoantibodies that bind with TSH receptors on thyroid cells, stimulating cell growth and function. Graves' hyperthyroidism occurs most commonly in the early to middle decades of life, while toxic multinodular goiter, thought to be the result of gradual overgrowth of autonomous thyroid cells, occurs at later ages, usually preceded by a history of nontoxic multinodular goiter. Less

Table 5–5. Causes of Hyperthyroidism

TSH Independent
  Diffuse toxic goiter (Graves' disease)
  Toxic multinodular goiter
  Solitary toxic nodule
  Thyroiditis (subacute or "painless")
  Iatrogenic or factitious

TSH Dependent
  Excessive placental hormones (hCG)
  TSH-secreting pituitary tumor

73

common forms include solitary toxic nodule and damage to the thyroid gland from thyroiditis, either subacute thyroiditis or so-called "painless thyrotoxic thyroiditis." The etiology of painless thyrotoxic thyroiditis is not known. There are features that suggest both autoimmune and infectious factors; it affects women much more commonly than men, and is often seen in the postpartum period.

Clinical Presentation

Hyperthyroidism is generally easier than hypothyroidism to diagnose on clinical grounds because the signs and symptoms are more apparent and more specific. These include rapid pulse, tremor, nervousness, weight loss, increased sweating, easy fatigue, and heat intolerance (Table 5–6). Thyroid enlargement is often but not invariably present; diffuse, symmetrical enlargement (sometimes with a bruit over the gland) is characteristic of Graves' disease, while an irregular, lobulated gland is seen with toxic multinodular goiter.

Diagnosis of Hyperthyroidism

With a sufficiently sensitive assay, TSH becomes an ideal test for hyperthyroidism as well as hypothyroidism. If TSH is normal (not suppressed), hyperthyroidism has been essentially

Table 5–6. Symptoms and Signs of Hyperthyroidism

Symptoms	Signs
Weight loss	Fine hair, thin skin
Fatigue	Onycholysis
Menstrual irregularities	Muscle weakness
Heat intolerance	Low cholesterol
Increased sweating	Glucose intolerance
Hyperdefecation	Tachycardia
Nervousness	Widened pulse pressure
Restlessness	Tremor, rapid DTRs
	Stare, lid lag

ruled out. If TSH is low, T_4 (or FT_4) and T_3 should be measured to determine the severity of hyperthyroidism. In hyperthyroidism, T_3 is often elevated earlier and to a greater degree than T_4. Combining the total T_3 measurement with a T_3 uptake ratio to calculate a free T_3 index (FT_3I) is helpful in adjusting the total T_3 for abnormalities in binding proteins.

The most conclusive test for hyperthyroidism is the TRH stimulation test (protocol, p. 218). High levels of thyroid hormone in the pituitary will block release of TSH. In a patient with equivocal symptoms of hyperthyroidism and T_4 or T_3 levels that are normal or slightly high, failure of TRH to stimulate a rise in TSH establishes the diagnosis of hyperthyroidism. This test, however, is not needed in most hyperthyroid patients and is rarely necessary now that sufficiently sensitive TSH assays are available.

Hyperthyroidism may be seen with normal total T_4 and FT_4 but an elevated T_3; this syndrome of "T_3 toxicosis" most commonly occurs following previous radioiodine treatment or surgical treatment for hyperthyroidism, or from treatment with thyroid hormone preparations that contain both T_4 and T_3. "T_4 toxicosis," high total T_4 and normal total T_3, is not a common situation. In many patients with high T_4 but low T_3 levels and clinical hyperthyroidism, the low T_3 is the result of the transient influence of drugs or stress. These patients will usually have high T_3 if tested again in a non-stressed state.

Determining the etiology of hyperthyroidism is important for deciding treatment. This may be possible on clinical grounds (e.g., Graves' disease with a diffuse goiter and exophthalmos; toxic multinodular goiter with known, long-standing multinodular thyroid enlargement; subacute thyroiditis with painful thyroid swelling and elevated sedimentation rate). Often, the clinical picture is not sufficiently clear to be confident of the etiology. Radioiodine uptake is useful, being negligible when the cause of hyperthyroidism is thyroiditis, moderately elevated (30 to 50% of administered dose at 24 hours) in toxic multinodular goiter, and markedly elevated (60% or higher) in most patients with Graves' hyperthyroidism. Thyroid uptake is needed to calculate a therapeutic dose of I-131. Thyroid scan adds helpful information in selected cases to distinguish toxic multinodular goiter from Graves' hyperthyroidism.

Thyroid stimulating immunoglobulins (TSI or TSAb) are antibodies that bind with the TSH receptor (TSAb) and stimulate thyroid cell function (TSI). Thyroid stimulating antibodies mediate the hyperthyroidism of Graves' disease and can be found in the serum of over 95% of patients with newly diagnosed Graves' disease. These antibodies bind with the TSH receptor and activate the same processes within the thyroid cell (hormone synthesis and cell growth) as does TSH itself. Other antibodies may occur that bind with the TSH receptor and block TSH action, leading to thyroid atrophy. Still other antibodies are involved in attracting chronic inflammatory cells to the thyroid and producing Hashimoto's thyroiditis. High titers of TSI may be passed from a pregnant mother to the fetus causing neonatal Graves' disease. There are conflicting studies regarding the prognostic significance of TSI. In most patients, measurement of TSI is not needed.

Accompanying the hyperthyroidism of Graves' disease in perhaps 10% of patients is moderate or severe *infiltrative ophthalmopathy*. There is infiltration of the extraocular muscles and retroorbital tissues with mucopolysaccharide material, probably mediated by antibodies. Usually, ophthalmopathy appears at about the same time that hyperthyroidism presents, but occasionally may precede or follow the hyperthyroidism by 12 to 18 months. Rarely, ophthalmopathy occurs without any abnormality in thyroid function ("euthyroid Graves' disease"). Thyroid ophthalmopathy may be more than a cosmetic problem, with forward protrusion of the eyes leading to exposure damage of the cornea, or pressure on the optic nerve leading to blindness. Management of mild to moderate ophthalmopathy is symptomatic (wetting agents); treatment of severe Graves' eye disease with steroids, orbital irradiation, or orbital decompression, should be left to centers with extensive experience with this problem.

Treatment of Hyperthyroidism

In most cases, *thyroiditis* causing hyperthyroidism is a self-limiting condition that will resolve in 4 to 12 weeks without residual thyroid function abnormality. If treatment is needed, beta-adrenergic blocking drugs are most useful in relieving the symptoms associated with increased adrenergic sensitivity (palpitations, nervousness, and tremor). Beta adrenergic blocking drugs may also be used for symptom relief in other forms of hyperthyroidism. Since hyperthyroid patients tend to be anxious and forgetful, choosing a drug that can be given once or twice a day like metoprolol (Lopressor) or nadolol (Corgard) will help with compliance.

There are several satisfactory choices for treating *Graves' hyperthyroidism,* but each has its drawbacks. Although remissions occur only in a minority of patients treated for 1 or 2 years with antithyroid drugs such as propylthiouracil (PTU) or methimazole (MMI, Tapazole), the proportion is substantial enough (30 to 40%) and the end result so desirable as to make this the first line of treatment. Even if destructive treatment (radioactive iodine or surgical) is chosen, stabilizing the patient first with antithyroid drugs makes the informed consent for treatment clearer and the course of treatment smoother. For mild or moderate disease, Tapazole is preferred to PTU because of its longer duration of action; 20 mg twice daily is a typical starting dose, with most patients becoming euthyroid in 4 to 8 weeks and then controlled with 20 mg once a day. Patients should be cautioned about the potentially serious development of leukopenia and instructed to discontinue their medication and have a blood count done at the first sign of infection (restarting their medication if the white blood count is normal).

Radioactive iodine or *surgical treatment* should be used for patients with Graves' disease who cannot be controlled with antithyroid drugs or who relapse after 12 to 24 months of treatment, as well as for patients with toxic multinodular goiter and solitary toxic nodules, conditions where remissions do not occur. Radioactive iodine in Graves' hyperthyroidism generally causes hypothyroidism to develop sooner (2 to 3 months after treatment) or later (hypothyroidism is less likely in toxic nodular goiter); hypothyroidism is so simple to treat that the trade seems worthwhile. There are no other significant complications from radioactive iodine treatment (no increase in malignancies, no problems with infertility or teratogenesis). Surgery has a lesser incidence of hypothyroidism than radioactive iodine, and significant complications are uncommon with an experienced surgeon; however, these complications are sufficiently serious (hypoparathyroidism, recurrent laryngeal nerve injury, anesthetic-related death) that radioactive iodine treatment is usually preferred to surgery.

Thyroid Storm

Thyroid storm is a rare but frequently fatal condition that can complicate almost any form of hyperthyroidism. Treatment is multifaceted: in addition to intravenous fluids, pressors, and other supportive measures, iodides are given to block the release of preformed hormone from the gland; PTU is given to block synthesis of new hormone (and preferred over Tapazole in severe hyperthyroidism because PTU also inhibits peripheral conversion of T_4 to T_3); beta-adrenergic blocking agents to reduce sympathetic overactivity (propranolol is preferred because it is the only beta antagonist that inhibits peripheral conversion of T_4 to T_3); other agents that block T_4 to T_3 conversion may also be added (glucocorticoids, ipodate); finally, for severe cases, plasmapheresis may be used to reduce the circulating levels of these protein bound hormones.

Cooper DS: Antithyroid drugs. N Engl J Med 1984; *311*:1353–1362.

Graham GD, Burman KD: Radioiodine treatment of Graves' disease: An assessment of its potential risks. Ann Intern Med 1986; *105*:900–905.

Hamburger JI: The autonomously functioning thyroid adenoma. N Engl J Med 1983; *309*:1512–1513.

Ivy HK, Wahner HW, Gorman CA: Triiodothyronine (T_3) toxicosis. Arch Intern Med 1971; *128*:529–539.

Jackson IMD: Hyper-thyroiditis–a diagnostic pitfall. N Engl J Med 1975; *293*:661–662.

Klein I, Levey GS: Silent thyrotoxic thyroiditis. Ann Intern Med 1982; *96*:242–244.

Nicoloff JT: Thyroid storm and myxedema coma. Med Clin North Am 1985; *69*:1005–1017.

Smith BR, McLachlan M, Furmaniak J: Autoantibodies to the thyrotropin receptor. Endocrine Reviews 1988; *9*:106–122.

Sugrue D, McEvoy M, Feely J, et al.: Hyperthyroidism in the land of Graves: Results of treatment by surgery, radioiodine and carbimazole in 837 cases. Quart J Med 1980; *193*:51–61.

Utiger RD: Beta-adrenergic-antagonist therapy for Graves' disease. N Engl J Med 1984; *310*:1597–1598.

NONTHYROID FACTORS AND THYROID TESTS: THE "EUTHYROID SICK" SYNDROME

Peripheral deiodination of T_4 is the primary source of T_3, the more potent of the two thyroid hormones. This enzymatic conversion is inhibited by a number of medications, by acute and chronic stress, and in a variety of acute and chronic non-thyroidal illnesses (Table 5–1). As conversion of T_4 to T_3 is reduced, conversion of T_4 to rT_3 increases, resulting in an increase of serum rT_3. Common test abnormalities accompanying nonthyroidal illnesses in euthyroid patients, the "euthyroid sick syndrome," (Table 5–7) include an increase in rT_3, lowering of total T_3 and FT_3I, and lowering of TBG and other binding protein levels. Low T_4 levels are often seen in sick euthyroid patients. Free T_4 may be high with acute illness or low with severe chronic illness. TSH and TRH responses are not usually affected (though transient elevation of TSH may be seen during recovery from nonthyroidal illness and TSH is suppressed by dopamine and large doses of glucocorticoids). Thus, in nonthyroidal ill-

Table 5–7. The Euthyroid Sick Syndrome: Changes in Thyroid Test Results

T_3 (RIA), low
rT_3, normal or high
T_4, FT_4I, normal or low
FT_4, normal, high, or low
Basal TSH, usually normal; may be low or high
TRH test, usually normal

ness, abnormal thyroid tests often are not indicative of thyroid disease. Hyperthyroid patients with acute or chronic nonthyroidal illness may have T_3 levels that are lowered into the normal range, and these patients sometimes show transient lowering of T_4 levels as well. TSH and TRH responses are usually valid despite nonthyroidal illness; these tests should be used if hyper- or hypothyroidism is suspected.

Hypothyroidism vs euthyroid sick. The most common dilemma presented by the test abnormalities seen with euthyroid sick syndrome occurs when hypothyroidism is suspected in an ill patient. T_3 is expected to be low in nonthyroidal illness and should not be measured for this purpose. If T_4 (or FT_4) is normal, hypothyroidism is most unlikely; however, low T_4 is often seen in the euthyroid sick. Serum TSH is probably the best single test to address the differential between euthyroid sick and hypothyroidism (in the absence of suspected pituitary or hypothalamic disease). A clear elevation of TSH (>30 μU/mL) would indicate hypothyroidism. Lesser TSH elevations may be seen transiently in euthyroid sick patients during recovery. However, dopamine or pharmacologic doses of glucocorticoids cause suppression of TSH and may result in a normal TSH in a hypothyroid patient. If the question of hypothyroidism cannot be resolved with TSH testing, measurement of reverse T_3 should help, rT_3 being low in hypothyroidism (either primary or secondary) and normal or high in euthyroid subjects.

Chopra IJ (moderator): Thyroid function in nonthyroidal illness. Ann Intern Med 1983; *98*:946–957.

Kaplan MM: Interactions between drugs and thyroid hormones. Thyroid Today 1981; *4/5*:1–6.

Kaplan MM, Larsen PR, Crantz FR, et al.: Prevalence of abnormal thyroid function test results in patients with acute medical illness. Am J Med 1982; *72*:9–16.

Utiger RD: Decreased extrathyroidal triiodothyronine production in nonthyroidal illness: benefit or harm? Am J Med 1980; *69*:807–810.

Wartofsky L, Burman KD: Alterations in thyroid function in patients with systemic illness: the "euthyroid sick" syndrome. Endocrine Reviews 1982; *3*:164–217.

EUTHYROID GOITER

Goiter is a generic term that means thyroid enlargement; a variety of benign and malignant thyroid conditions may present as goiter. Goiters may be diffuse or with single or multiple nodules. Some of these conditions may affect thyroid function, causing either hyper- or hypothyroidism; serum TSH or other thyroid function test should be done to exclude one of these disorders. If physical examination suggests a localized abnormality, fine needle aspiration for cytology should be considered. The main causes of euthyroid goiter are Hashimoto's thyroiditis, (nontoxic) multinodular goiter, and "simple" euthyroid goiter. While some authorities suggest further work-up before treatment, others suggest no evaluation or treatment (which seems appropriate for patients with small goiters). Since some of these goiters will enlarge without treatment, and suppressing TSH with L-thyroxine treatment will prevent enlargement, a practical approach is to prescribe suppressive doses of L-thyroxine (remembering that perhaps 10% of patients with multinodular goiter have nonsuppressible function and will become hyperthyroid with additional thyroid hormone), and continuing treatment and periodic (yearly) observation lifelong. Further studies such as antimicrosomal antibodies and thyroid scans before and after suppression may be useful in selected cases.

THYROID NODULES

Background, Pathophysiology

Nodular thyroid disease is common; the prevalence is approximately 2 to 4%. Solitary or dominant thyroid nodules are usually due to one of several benign thyroid conditions (a dominant nodule is a discrete area of nodularity in a multinodular thyroid gland). However, thyroid carcinoma is found in 10 to 15% of patients with thyroid nodules, so the possibility that a nodule might represent thyroid malignancy must not be overlooked. Figure 5–4 shows an estimate of the relative frequency of the different disorders that may present as nodular thyroid disease. Nonthyroidal conditions that sometimes present as a thyroid nodule include thyroid abscess, cervical lipoma, and metastatic carcinoma.

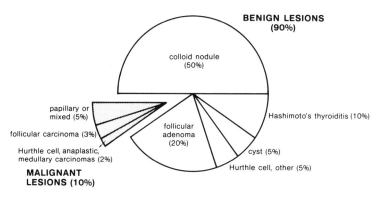

Fig. 5–4. Causes of solitary thyroid nodules. (Used with permission from Watts NB: Lessons from a patient with a solitary thyroid nodule. Emory U J Med 1988; *2*:64–70.

Clinical Presentation

Most thyroid nodules are detected coincidentally by primary physicians, although occasionally, nodules are noted by friends, family members, or the patient as a visible or palpable bulge in the neck. These nodules are usually too small to produce local symptoms (e.g., pressure, pain, dysphagia); rarely, rapid enlargement or hoarseness occur. Most patients with thyroid nodules have normal thyroid gland function, so signs and symptoms of thyroid hormone excess or deficiency are unlikely to be present. Goals in the evaluation and therapy of a patient with a solitary or dominant thyroid nodule include early diagnosis and treatment of thyroid malignancies while minimizing the need for surgery for the diagnosis of benign disease.

Diagnosis of Thyroid Nodules

Proper physical examination of the thyroid requires a great deal of practice; nodules <1 cm in diameter are easily missed. In addition to examining the patient in the seated position, it is helpful to examine the thyroid gland with the patient supine and their neck gently hyperextended by a pillow. The outline of the nodule can be traced on the skin with a ballpoint pen and the tracing transferred to paper to be kept as a permanent record in the patient's chart, providing an objective measurement of nodule size for future reference.

Fine needle aspiration (FNA) for cytology is the single most helpful test to decide if a nodule is malignant or not. The procedure is simple and almost painless. Most benign and malignant conditions can be promptly and accurately identified. Needle puncture will determine whether a lesion is cystic or solid (eliminating the need for thyroid ultrasound). In 1 to 2% of aspirations there is insufficient cytologic material for diagnosis, though this can usually be remedied by repeat aspiration. False positive results are seen in approximately 3 to 5% of cases, and false negatives in 1 to 2%. Availability of FNA is limited by the lack of trained persons to do the aspiration (a simple technique to master, but one that requires continuing experience to maintain adequacy) and the availability of skilled cytopathologists to interpret the samples.

For proper application of thyroid cytology, interpretation is important. In addition to "benign" and "malignant" cytologies, it is useful to consider an "indeterminant" group, where the cells appear benign but malignancy can not be excluded with certainty without histologic examination of the nodule. Follicular and Hurthle cell neoplasms comprise this group; most are benign, but histologic evidence of malignancy (tumor invasion of the capsule, blood vessels, or lymphatics) may be present with no diagnostic abnormality in the cells themselves. We use the categories "follicular neoplasm" and "Hurthle cell neoplasm" to indicate this indeterminate category, where the diagnosis or exclusion of malignancy must be made by surgery.

Certain findings on *physical examination* are suggestive of thyroid malignancy: large size (>3.5 cm in diameter), hard consistency, fixation to surrounding tissues, associated lymphadenopathy and vocal cord paralysis, all indicate a high risk for thyroid cancer. Benign nodules are more common in women between the ages of 25 and 55, so malignancy is more likely in males and at extremes of age (<25 or >55). A history of external irradiation exposure to the head or neck area indicates an increased risk of thyroid neoplasia; thyroid nodules are found in 20 to 30% of such patients, and 20 to 30% of these nodules will be malignant. Family history of medullary carcinoma of the thyroid or multiple endocrine neoplasia syndrome is quite significant, but these conditions are rare.

Blood tests of thyroid hormones or thyrotropin (T_4, T_3, TSH) should be done in all patients with nodular thyroid disease. Elevated levels of T_4 and T_3 would suggest a toxic nodule, a condition that is almost always benign. A high TSH, indicating thyroid gland failure, can be seen with multinodular goiter or with Hashimoto's thyroiditis; both conditions may present with asymmetric enlargement of the thyroid that gives the appearance of nodularity. Antithyroglobulin or antimicrosomal antibodies are typically elevated in patients with Hashimoto's thyroiditis; however, Hashimoto's disease is common and may be present in patients who also have coincidental thyroid neoplasia. Serum levels of thyroglobulin are elevated in most patients with well-differentiated thyroid carcinoma; since thyroglobulin levels are also elevated in a variety of benign thyroid conditions, this test cannot be relied on in the differential diagnosis of a specific nodule. Serum calcitonin is almost always elevated in patients with medullary carcinoma of the thyroid and is quite important in evaluating patients with a family history of multiple endocrine neoplasia syndrome. Since medullary carcinoma of the thyroid is quite rare, calcitonin measurements are not useful in the routine evaluation of patients with solitary thyroid nodules.

Thyroid scans have long served as the next diagnostic step after history, physical examination, and routine blood tests. If a nodule is "hot" on scan (that is, greater uptake of isotope in the nodule than in the surrounding tissue), there is a low probability of malignancy. However, over 90% of solitary thyroid nodules are "cold," and variations in "coolness" or "warmness" are not helpful in diagnosis. Thyroid scans are expensive, and it is not cost effective to do a scan in every patient to detect the occasional "hot" nodule. Thyroid scans can be useful in selected patients, for example, when physical examination is difficult or when hyperfunction is suggested by blood tests, but routine scanning of all patients with thyroid nodules should be abandoned.

Thyroid ultrasonography can detect small, nonpalpable nodules. Even though a nodule seems to be solitary by palpation, ultrasound may reveal a multinodular goiter, providing some reassurance that the nodule is benign. In most patients, however, the size of the nodule in question can be determined by physical examination, and the presence of multiple nodules, while reassuring, does not exclude malignancy. Thyroid ultrasound is 90 to 95% accurate in determining whether a nodule is solid, cystic, or mixed. Though a mixed cystic-solid lesion may well be a degenerating neoplasm, most authorities agree that thyroid carcinoma is unlikely in a purely cystic lesion. If a needle aspiration of the nodule is to be done, the nature of the nodule (solid vs cystic vs mixed) can be determined with greater accuracy and with less expense than by ultrasound. For these reasons, routine ultrasound of thyroid nodules is not recommended.

Suppressive therapy with thyroid hormone is based on the assumption that when pituitary secretion of TSH is suppressed by administration of thyroid hormone, benign nodules get smaller (and sometimes disappear) while malignant lesions will not change or will increase in size. However, occasional cancers will shrink with suppressive therapy, and about 50% of benign nodules will not change in size; only about 10% of thyroid nodules actually disappear on suppression. Suppressive therapy is of limited use in the initial diagnostic evaluation; it remains helpful for following patients with benign cytologic findings or to reduce the risk of recurrent nodularity after surgery for benign nodular disease, and is a critical part of the management after surgery for well-differentiated thyroid carcinoma.

Treatment of Thyroid Nodules

Recommendations for treatment can be based on the cytologic diagnosis, as shown in Figure 5–5. Most patients with well-differentiated thyroid carcinoma are identified promptly and surgery can be done without unnecessary delay for other diagnostic tests. Patients whose cytologic diagnosis is a benign disorder (e.g., colloid nodule, Hashimoto's thyroiditis) should

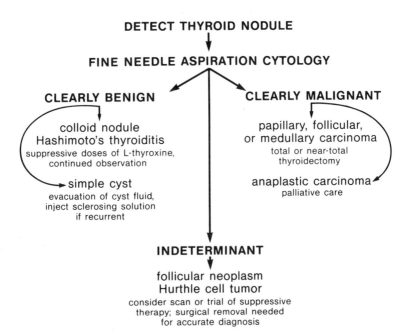

Fig. 5–5. Approach to the management of solitary thyroid nodules based on cytologic findings. (Used with permission from Watts NB: Lessons from a patient with a solitary thyroid nodule. Emory U J Med 1988; 2:64–70.)

be placed on L-thyroxine suppressive therapy to prevent further growth of the nodule and are followed indefinitely, rechecked in 2 to 3 months, then 6 months, then yearly. For the rare patient whose nodule increases in size despite suppressive therapy, reaspiration or surgery should be done. Patients with purely cystic nodules are usually cured by the initial aspiration; cysts that reaccumulate should be reaspirated, and, if recurrent after a second or third aspiration, injected with a sclerosing solution such as tetracycline.

Surgical excision may be necessary if a benign nodule is large enough to cause cosmetic or mechanical problems or if the patient remains apprehensive despite a reassuring cytology. Where malignancy cannot be excluded on cytologic grounds ("follicular neoplasm"), surgery is advised.

Ashcraft MW, Van Herle AJ: Management of thyroid nodules. I: History and physical examination, blood tests, x-ray tests, and ultrasonography. Head Neck Surg 1981; 3:216–230.

Ashcraft MW, Van Herle AJ: Management of thyroid nodules. II: Scanning techniques, thyroid suppressive therapy, and fine needle aspiration. Head Neck Surg 1981; 3:297–322.

Rojeski MT, Gharib H: Nodular thyroid disease: Evaluation and management. N Engl J Med 1985; 313:428–435.

Van Herle AJ (moderator): The thyroid nodule. Ann Intern Med 1982; 96:221–232.

Watts NB: Solitary thyroid nodules: An overview, with emphasis on fine needle aspiration cytology. J Med Assoc Ga 1985; 74:710–714.

Watts NB: Lessons from a patient with a solitary thyroid nodule. Emory U J Med 1988; 2:64–70.

THYROID CARCINOMA

Background, Pathophysiology

Primary carcinomas of the thyroid occur in several varieties: (1) well-differentiated malignancies of thyroid follicular cells (follicular, papillary, or mixed), (2) malignancies of the calcitonin-producing C-cells of the thyroid (medullary carcinoma), and (3) anaplastic carcinoma.

The most common type of thyroid malignancy is well-differentiated carcinoma of the thyroid. These malignancies may occur at any age and affect women twice as commonly as men. External irradiation to the head or neck area in infancy, childhood, or adolescence is a risk factor for this type of thyroid neoplasia; about 30% of subjects at risk develop nodular thyroid disease, and 20 to 30% of the nodules are malignant. In the 1940s and 1950s, radiation treatment was commonly given to infants for enlargement of the thymus, to children for tonsillitis, and to adolescents for acne. Low doses (up to 600 mrem) given during the time of growth appear to predispose to thyroid neoplasia for up to 40 years later. Radiation-induced malignancies are no more aggressive than those that arise de novo. Some authorities consider papillary carcinoma to be less aggressive than the follicular variety; papillary tumors are more likely to recur locally and the follicular variant is more prone to hematogenous spread. In practice, this distinction does not appear to have much importance, and many well-differentiated thyroid carcinomas contain elements of both papillary and follicular forms.

Medullary carcinoma of the thyroid is less common than well-differentiated carcinoma. Most of these tumors also arise de novo, though perhaps 10% are seen in families affected with multiple endocrine neoplasia type IIa (medullary carcinoma of the thyroid, hyperparathyroidism, and pheochromocytoma) or type IIb (medullary carcinoma of the thyroid, pheochromocytoma, and mucocutaneous neurofibromas).

There are no definite risk factors for anaplastic carcinoma of the thyroid; there is some evidence that external irradiation to well-differentiated tumors may predispose to anaplastic degeneration.

Clinical Presentation

The usual presentation for well-differentiated thyroid carcinoma is an asymptomatic mass, a solitary thyroid nodule. Evaluation of the solitary thyroid nodule has been discussed. Most cases of medullary carcinoma and anaplastic carcinoma also present as a mass, the latter often with signs and symptoms of local invasion. There is no humoral syndrome associated with these tumors.

Diagnosis of Thyroid Carcinoma

Thyroid carcinoma may be suspected preoperatively based on fine needle aspiration, but the final diagnosis requires surgical excision, which is also part of appropriate treatment. Patients who are at risk for medullary carcinoma may be identified early by way of a stimulation test, where calcitonin is measured after administration of a provocative agent (the combination of calcium and pentagastrin seems more sensitive than either alone) (protocol, p. 207).

Treatment of Thyroid Carcinoma

Anaplastic carcinoma is usually fatal in less than a year after diagnosis, so treatment should be palliative only.

Medullary carcinoma is a slow-growing, locally invasive tumor. It does not respond well to radiation or chemotherapy, so attempted total radical excision is warranted, even if other structures in the neck must be sacrificed.

Long-term survival from *well-differentiated thyroid carcinoma* is good, approaching over 90% with proper treatment. There is some question regarding ideal treatment for papillary and follicular carcinomas; some authorities favor limited surgery (subtotal thyroidectomy) and reserve radioactive iodine treatment for selected cases. Most authorities favor a standardized approach that includes near-total thyroidectomy (leaving behind a small amount of posterior capsule to protect the parathyroids and recurrent nerves) and ablation of the thyroid remnant 6 weeks after surgery with 100 mCi of I-131. Routine radical neck dissection is *not* indicated for well-differentiated thyroid carcinoma.

Regardless of the extent of surgery and use of radioactive iodine, a sufficient dose of L-thyroxine should be given to suppress TSH, since TSH is a growth factor for normal and neoplastic thyroid cells. The suppressive dose is slightly higher than the replacement dose (average is 0.1 μg L-thyroxine per pound of body weight per day); adequacy of the dose should be assessed by a TRH stimulation test (protocol, p. 218) or highly sensitive TSH assay. T_4 or FT_4 should also be done to be certain that the dose is not excessive.

Follow-up of patients with thyroid carcinoma should include at least yearly TSH and T_4 measurements as well as careful examination for local recurrences. If the thyroid remnant has been ablated, total body I-131 scans can be done (generally at 1, 3, and 5 years after surgery and every 5 years afterwards). Patients must be off L-thyroxine for 6 weeks prior to scanning; T_3 (Cytomel) 25 μg three times daily may be substituted for 4 weeks to minimize the time the patient is hypothyroid, then all thyroid hormone stopped for 2 weeks before the scan. Serum thyroglobulin should be low once all thyroid tissue is removed. Some authorities feel that thyroglobulin measurements may be substituted for the scan in low-risk patients, with an elevated or rising thyroglobulin level indicating probable recurrent disease. Recurrences are treated with surgical excision when possible, with I-131, or external radiation if the recurrent tumor does not take up radioactive iodine.

Beierwaltes WH: Controversies in the treatment of thyroid cancer: The University of Michigan approach. Thyroid Today 1983; 6:1–5.

Leeper R: Controversies in the treatment of thyroid cancer: The New York Memorial Hospital approach. Thyroid Today 1982; 5:1–4.

Mazzaferri EL, Young RL: Papillary thyroid carcinoma: A 10 year follow-up report of the impact of therapy in 576 patients. Am J Med 1981; 70:511–518.

Saaman NA, Mahewhwari YK, Nader S, et al.: Impact of therapy for differentiated carcinoma of the thyroid: An analysis of 706 cases. J Clin Endocrinol Metab 1983; 56:1131–1138.

Sarkar SD, Beierwaltes WH, Gill SP, et al.: Subsequent fertility and birth histories of children and adolescents treated with ^{131}I for thyroid cancer. J Nucl Med 1976; 17:460–464.

Schlumberger M, Tubiana M, De Vathaire F, et al.: Long term results of treatment of 283 patients with lung and bone metastases from differentiated thyroid carcinoma. J Clin Endocrinol Metab 1986; 63:960–967.

Schneider AB, Recant W, Pinsky SM, et al.: Radiation-induced thyroid carcinoma: Clinical course and results of therapy in 296 patients. Ann Intern Med 1986; 105:405–412.

THYROIDITIS

Background, Pathophysiology

Inflammation of the thyroid gland is known as thyroiditis. There are several forms. Hashimoto's thyroiditis is an autoimmune disorder which affects approximately 1% of the population. It is more common in people with other autoimmune diseases (Graves' hyperthyroidism, type I diabetes mellitus, pernicious anemia, etc.) and is associated with certain HLA types (DR5, B8). Females are affected 8 times more frequently than males. Subacute thyroiditis is thought to be of viral etiology and has a prevalence of 0.1%, with no sexual predominance. Alterations of thyroid function may be seen with both. "Painless thyrotoxic thyroiditis" has been discussed under hyperthyroidism. Rare forms of thyroiditis (Reidel's, DeQuervain's, bacterial) must be mentioned for completeness but are too infrequent to merit more discussion here.

Clinical Presentation

Hashimoto's thyroiditis (also known as chronic lymphocytic thyroiditis) has a varied presentation and clinical course. Classically the presentation is a euthyroid patient with a symmetrically enlarged, firm and "bosselated" goiter; eventually, the thyroid gland is destroyed by the inflammatory reaction and hypothyroidism develops. However, some patients with Hashimoto's thyroiditis have an acute or subacute presentation with local pain and tenderness and systemic symptoms. The goiter may be asymmetric or have the appearance of a solitary nodule. Hypothyroidism does not always develop, and even when it does, it may be transient rather than permanent. While Hashimoto's thyroiditis does not usually cause hyperthyroidism, it is found coincidentally in approximately 20% of patients with Graves' hyperthyroidism. With regard to thyroid function, there is initially a defect of organification of iodine which is manifest as an increase in the uptake (but not retention) of radioactive iodine by the gland at a time when thyroid hormone production (and circulating thyroid hormone levels) are normal or even low. Many patients with Hashimoto's thyroiditis have only a small goiter and a nonprogressive course.

Subacute thyroiditis has a fairly abrupt onset of systemic symptoms including fever, malaise and myalgias, usually accompanied by pain, redness, and swelling over the thyroid. While circulating levels of thyroid hormones are often elevated as the result of release of preformed hormone from damaged thyroid follicles, signs and symptoms of hyperthyroidism are often overshadowed by systemic symptoms. Subacute thyroiditis may be without systemic symptoms but with pain, usually in the thyroid and radiating to the neck or angle of the jaw, but sometimes as mysterious pain in the jaw with few or no signs or symptoms to point to the thyroid.

Diagnosis of Thyroiditis

Hashimoto's thyroiditis often can be diagnosed by the clinical picture alone. If additional confirmation is needed, titers of antimicrosomal antibodies are elevated in over 90% of patients (antithyroglobulin antibodies are usually elevated also, but add little or no diagnostic information to antimicrosomal antibody titers). Fine needle biopsy of the thyroid can also be done. TSH or other test of thyroid function should be done.

Subacute thyroiditis is diagnosed on clinical grounds. There is always a striking elevation of erythrocyte sedimentation rate (>60 mm/h) in active disease. TSH or other test of thyroid hormone status should be done; the typical evolution is for high levels of thyroid hormones and low TSH to be found initially, progressing to hypothyroid values before returning spontaneously to normal over 8 to 12 weeks.

Treatment of Thyroiditis

Pain in the thyroid should be treated symptomatically, initially with antiinflammatory doses of salicylates, then, if needed, with nonsteroidal antiinflammatory drugs, and finally, if significant pain and discomfort persist, with glucocorticoids. Salicylates are also useful for the systemic manifestations of subacute thyroiditis.

Thyroid enlargement from thyroiditis is usually not sufficient to cause cosmetic or local concerns, and the enlargement from subacute thyroiditis usually regresses without treatment. Some patients with Hashimoto's thyroiditis will require suppressive doses of L-thyroxine to prevent undesirable enlargement, while patients with a small goiter and normal thyroid function may simply be followed.

Thyroid dysfunction associated with subacute thyroiditis rarely requires treatment, though beta-adrenergic blocking agents may be needed in some patients during the early stages. It is best to withhold thyroid hormone treatment later in the evolution of subacute thyroiditis, since permanent hypothyroidism is uncommon. The decision regarding when to begin thyroid hormone replacement for Hashimoto's thyroiditis is not always simple; in general, the patient with symptoms of hypothyroidism and/or a TSH >20 µU/mL should be started on L-thyroxine. Even though thyroid dysfunction is occasionally transient in Hashimoto's thyroiditis, it is usually best to continue treatment lifelong.

Hay ID: Thyroiditis: A clinical update. Mayo Clin Proc 1985; *60*:836–843.

Hamburger JI: The various presentations of thyroiditis: Diagnostic considerations. Ann Intern Med 1986; *104*:219–224.

Tunbridge WMG, Brewis M, French JM, et al.: Natural history of autoimmune thyroiditis. Br Med J 1981; *282*:258–262.

6

Adrenal Cortex

ADRENAL GLANDS

Introduction, Background, Physiology

Three main classes of hormones are produced by the adrenal cortex: (1) glucocorticoids, (2) mineralocorticoids, and (3) adrenal androgens. Glucocorticoids are named because of their influence on glucose homeostasis, but glucocorticoids also affect intermediary metabolism of protein and fat, immunity, healing, regulation of blood pressure, and the response to stress. Cortisol is the most important in man. Mineralocorticoids influence sodium and potassium exchange by the kidney and play a major part in the regulation of extracellular volume. Aldosterone is the most important mineralocorticoid in man. The role of adrenal androgens (such as androstenedione and dehydroepiandrosterone) in normal physiology is not well understood.

Adrenocorticotropic hormone (ACTH) is produced by the pituitary gland and controls secretion of glucocorticoids and adrenal androgens (mineralocorticoid secretion is regulated by the renin-angiotensin system). ACTH production, in turn, is stimulated by corticotropin releasing hormone (CRH), which is produced by the hypothalamus (Fig. 6–1). Normally, secretion of ACTH is coordinated with the sleep-wake cycle, with highest values between 06:00–08:00 and lowest between 22:00–02:00. Levels of cortisol follow and parallel those of ACTH. This pattern, called "diurnal" or "circadian" rhythm, is reversed in individuals who operate on unconventional sleep-wake schedules (e.g., "graveyard" shifts). In addition to changing with diurnal rhythm, cortisol is secreted episodically, with two- to three-fold fluctuations in serum concentration occurring over 20 to 30 minutes.

As with many endocrine systems, the hypothalamic-pituitary-adrenal axis involves regulation by feedback. Lowering the level of cortisol causes a rise in ACTH secretion; increasing

91

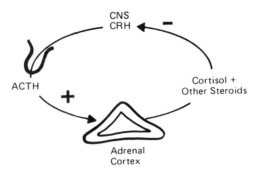

Fig. 6–1. Hypothalamic-pituitary-adrenal axis.

levels of glucocorticoid inhibit release of ACTH from the pituitary. However, this negative feedback can be overcome by stress, one of the primary stimuli for release of CRH. ACTH and cortisol normally increase during physical or emotional stress. The degree of this increase depends on the duration and intensity of the stress. During uncomplicated acute infections, plasma cortisol may increase up to six times normal. Diurnal variation is lost when stress is prolonged and severe.

Biochemistry

Cortisol circulates in blood ~80% bound to a carrier protein, cortisol-binding globulin (CBG); only the free (non-protein-bound) fraction is biologically active. High or low concentrations of CBG may be inherited or acquired (e.g., increased CBG is seen with estrogen treatment or pregnancy, decreases are seen with androgen treatment or nephrotic syndrome). Changes in the concentration of this binding protein, while not of physiologic importance, can confuse the interpretation of cortisol measurements in blood. An increased level of CBG results in a higher total plasma cortisol level for a given level of free (active) cortisol, and a decreased level of CBG leads to a low total cortisol but a normal free level.

Cortisol is metabolized to inactive compounds in peripheral tissues (primarily the liver), mainly to glucuronide and sulfate conjugates, 17-hydroxysteroids, and 17-ketogenic steroids. Cortisol and its metabolites are excreted by the kidneys. Excretion of 17-hydroxysteroids and 17-ketosteroids reflects cortisol production, but is also influenced by body mass and other variables; measurement of these compounds largely has been superseded by specific cortisol determinations. Urinary free cortisol ("free" refers to freely filtered and not conjugated) correlates well with cortisol production rate and is not significantly influenced by body mass.

Sensitive and specific assays for cortisol are available in kit form and are widely used. While cortisol can be measured by a variety of methods, including colorimetry, fluorometry, and HPLC, most current assays rely on immunoassay techniques.

ADRENAL INSUFFICIENCY

Background, Pathophysiology

Glucocorticoid deficiency results in a constellation of non-specific and sometimes subtle signs and symptoms: easy fatigue, weakness, postural dizziness, postural hypotension, nausea, and loss of appetite. Hyponatremia may occur due to inability of the kidneys to excrete a maximally dilute urine in the absence of glucocorticoids. Combined deficiency of glucocorticoids and mineralocorticoids leads to more severe hypotension, hyponatremia, and hyperkalemia. Also, ACTH secretion from the pituitary gland is markedly increased in primary adrenal insufficiency, leading to hyperpigmentation of the skin and mucous membranes through melanocyte-stimulating activity.

Clinical Presentation

Deficient function of the adrenal cortex may cause significant morbidity and, when severe, may cause death. Fortunately, adrenal deficiency states are uncommon; however, signs and symptoms suggestive of adrenal insufficiency (e.g., fatigue, weakness, dizziness) are commonly seen in the absence of adrenal disease. A high level of suspicion is necessary to make the diagnosis in early or mild cases. A variety of diagnostic tests can be used to "rule-in" or "rule-out" adrenal insufficiency, but selective use of these tests is needed to minimize unnecessary expense.

Adrenal insufficiency is termed primary when it results from diseases of the adrenal gland. *Primary adrenal insufficiency,* also known as *Addison's disease,* most commonly is due to adrenal destruction by autoimmune processes, but may also be caused by hemorrhage, infections (including tuberculosis and fungal infections), or metastatic malignancy. Since the entire adrenal cortex is destroyed in primary adrenal insufficiency, all classes of adrenal hormones are deficient. Patients have signs and symptoms of both glucocorticoid and mineralocorticoid

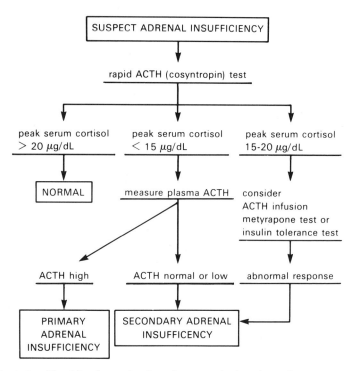

Fig. 6–2. Algorithm for evaluation of suspected adrenal insufficiency.

deficiency, as well as ACTH excess, which in fully established cases include hyperpigmentation of the skin and mucous membranes; dehydration with hypotension, hyponatremia, and hyperkalemia; weakness; nausea; and anorexia.

Secondary adrenal insufficiency results from abnormalities of the pituitary or hypothalamus such as primary or metastatic tumors, inflammatory or ischemic insults. However, the most common cause of secondary adrenal insufficiency is iatrogenic: prior treatment with pharmacologic doses of glucocorticoids that suppress pituitary ACTH release, leading to adrenal atrophy. Glucocorticoid deficiency occurs with both primary and secondary adrenal insufficiency. Mineralocorticoid deficiency and ACTH excess are not seen with secondary adrenal insufficiency. In secondary adrenal insufficiency, mineralocorticoid secretion is maintained in the absence of ACTH through the renin-angiotensin system. Secondary adrenal insufficiency is usually more subtle in its presentation than the primary form; hypotension is less severe, and hyperkalemia and hyperpigmentation are not seen. Except in patients previously treated with glucocorticoids, isolated ACTH deficiency is uncommon; secondary adrenal insufficiency due to structural lesions of the pituitary or hypothalamus is usually accompanied by hypogonadism and hypothyroidism.

Both primary and secondary adrenal insufficiency may be complete or partial; the severity of the clinical manifestations depends on the extent of the hormone deficiency.

Diagnosis of Adrenal Insufficiency

In severe cases of adrenal insufficiency the diagnosis is usually easy to confirm. A low serum cortisol in the face of an elevated ACTH level indicates primary adrenal insufficiency, where a low cortisol with a low or inappropriately "normal" level of ACTH indicates secondary adrenal insufficiency. In an emergency situation, where it seems prudent to institute treatment with glucocorticoids immediately, it should be possible prior to treatment to draw a blood sample to be assayed later for cortisol and ACTH to establish the diagnosis. Even then, the use of dexamethasone (a potent glucocorticoid analog that will not interfere with cortisol determination) permits more definitive testing (such as the rapid ACTH test, protocol p. 207).

In early or mild cases of adrenal insufficiency, when the diagnosis is not obvious, a groping approach to test ordering often confuses the issues.

Cortisol Determinations: Serum or Urine? Serum cortisol concentration is affected by a number of factors including the level of cortisol binding globulin, time of day (diurnal variation), and episodic secretion. Urinary free cortisol more accurately reflects cortisol secretion than does a single serum measurement. This is extremely important in the diagnosis of suspected adrenocortical excess states (Cushing's syndrome). A few investigators have suggested that urinary cortisol determinations are useful in the evaluation of suspected adrenal insufficiency but, partly because of longer experience and partly because of ease of sampling, serum cortisol determination is preferred to urinary measurement for evaluation of adrenal reserve as long as proper conditions are met.

Serum Cortisol Determination: Basal, Random, or Stimulated? While a normal AM serum cortisol level makes a diagnosis of adrenal insufficiency unlikely, there remains the possibility that adrenal responsiveness to stress might be impaired despite adequate basal cortisol production. Since cortisol levels vary throughout the day and the magnitude of the cortisol response to stress is unpredictable, basal or random cortisol determinations have limited value.

Testing Adrenal Responsiveness. If the adrenal glands have been regularly stimulated by ACTH there should be prompt and significant rise in serum cortisol with acute ACTH stimulation. A simple stimulation test is recommended for screening purposes (protocol p. 207). *Cosyntropin* (Cortrosyn, Organon Pharmaceuticals) is the 1–24 amino acid sequence of ACTH and has a brief half-life and rapid onset of action. If a patient has a normal baseline serum cortisol and an appropriate peak serum cortisol after cosyntropin administration, one can be quite confident that primary adrenal insufficiency has been excluded, and, with rare exceptions, normal results indicate integrity of the hypothalamic-pituitary-adrenal axis.

The *cosyntropin test (rapid ACTH test)* can be done in a variety of ways. After a baseline sample for cortisol has been obtained, cosyntropin is given intramuscularly or intravenously in a dose of 250 μg. For screening purposes, to "rule-out" adrenal insufficiency, a single additional sample 30, 45, or 60 minutes after injection is adequate; when adrenal insufficiency is strongly suspected, most authorities prefer three samples: baseline, 30 minutes, and 60 minutes. Various criteria have been recommended for interpretation that include specific incremental rises as well as absolute peak values. A peak cortisol level ≥20 μg/dL is a good indicator of normal adrenal function, but it is reassuring to also see a rise of ≥7 μg/dL above the baseline level.

Patients with an abnormal response in the rapid ACTH test deserve further study. An elevated *plasma ACTH* in a patient with a subnormal response to cosyntropin indicates primary adrenal insufficiency. No additional diagnostic tests would be needed to establish the diagnosis (though further studies might be needed to establish the etiology). If the cortisol response to cosyntropin stimulation is subnormal and plasma ACTH is low or "normal," secondary adrenal insufficiency must be tested for. To prove that the adrenal glands are able to respond to ACTH stimulation, an infusion of cosyntropin (500 μg in 1000 mL of 0.9% saline solution given over 4 hours) should cause an increase of serum cortisol to >20 μg/dL.

Testing the Hypothalamic-Pituitary-Adrenal Axis. Assuming that the adrenal glands can respond to ACTH stimulation, the integrity of the hypothalamic-pituitary-adrenal axis can then be tested in a variety of ways. The most reliable test is also the most complicated and most risky to perform: the insulin tolerance test (protocol p. 214). The stress of insulin-induced hypoglycemia provokes an increase in ACTH from the pituitary gland, which in turn causes an increase in cortisol secretion. Insulin-induced hypoglycemia is somewhat dangerous, so this test should only be done with an experienced physician in attendance. The test is performed by giving Regular insulin, 0.1 to 0.15 Units/kg intravenously; samples are drawn for glucose and cortisol at baseline and every 30 mintues for 90 minutes. A rise of serum cortisol to >20 μg/dL is a normal response if the patient was adequately stressed, as shown by definite symptoms of hypoglycemia or a blood glucose level <40 mg/dL.

The hypothalamic-pituitary-adrenal axis may also be tested by giving metyrapone, a drug that inhibits the enzymatic step preceding the synthesis of cortisol (protocol p. 216). The fall in cortisol induced by metyrapone provokes a rise in ACTH from the pituitary gland, leading to stimulation of adrenal synthesis of cortisol precursors, specifically 11-deoxycortisol (compound S), which can be measured in blood. As a simple outpatient test, metyrapone 3.0 g is given orally at bedtime and plasma 11-deoxycortisol and cortisol are measured the next morning. Plasma 11-deoxycortisol <7 μg/dL with a serum cortisol <3 μg/dL indicates secondary adrenal insufficiency. A more formal approach is to give metyrapone 750 mg orally every 4 hours for 24 hours and measure urinary 17-hydroxysteroids the day before, the day of metyrapone administration, and the day after. Comparing the day after metyrapone administration to a baseline day, a threefold increase of urinary 17-hydroxysteroids, reflecting the buildup of cortisol precursors, is considered a normal response.

In the future, testing of the hypothalamic-pituitary-adrenal axis may be simplified by the availability of corticotropin-releasing hormone (CRH) for diagnostic use. This peptide hormone can be administered intravenously and the response of ACTH and cortisol to a bolus injection measured.

Treatment of Adrenal Insufficiency

Glucocorticoid replacement should mimic the natural cycles insofar as is possible. Long-acting glucocorticoid analogs such as dexamethasone are not satisfactory for maintenance replacement since their long duration of action results in lack of diurnal variation. Synthetic glucocorticoids such as prednisone and methylprednisolone do not offer any advantages over hydrocortisone or cortisone acetate. Hydrocortisone is the same as cortisol; cortisone acetate is converted to cortisol for activity. Average replacement for basal (nonstressed) circumstances is hydrocortisone 20 mg each morming and 10 mg each afternoon (or cortisone acetate 25 mg each morning and 12.5 mg each afternoon). There are several caveats regarding glucocorticoid replacement:

1. Be certain to give the second dose in the afternoon, not at bedtime; postponing the second dose until bedtime usually results in fatigue in the afternoon and psychologic stimulation at bedtime.
2. Be certain to inform patients of the need to continue medication lifelong and to increase their dose in times of stress. A good rule of thumb is to triple the maintenance dose for 3 days for mild or moderate stress; up to 100 mg every 8 hours is recommended for severe stress such as surgery under general anesthesia.
3. Be certain that patients know to get an injection of steroid if they are unable to take medication by mouth; the combination of the stress of illness and failure or inability to take replacement steroids often leads to rapid deterioration, even death.
4. Be certain patients have identification showing adrenal insufficiency (wallet card, necklace, or bracelet).

Assessment of the adequacy of glucocorticoid treatment is largely based on clinical assessment. If signs of Cushing's syndrome appear, the dose should be reduced. If hypotension, fatigue, and weakness are present, the dose should be increased. Serum cortisol levels are not useful, since these drugs have only a brief half-life in the circulation. Urine free cortisol or 17-hydroxysteroids may give a rough indication of replacement in patients taking hydrocortisone or cortisone acetate (but not other steroids), but these parameters have not been well studied. In patients with primary adrenal insufficiency, plasma ACTH measurements may be useful as a guide to adequate replacement therapy, being high if the patient is undertreated and suppressed if overtreated.

It is usually necessary to add *mineralocorticoid replacement* for patients with primary adrenal insufficiency. Fludrohydrocortisone (Florinef), 0.1 or 0.2 mg daily, is usually adequate. The dose can be monitored by following arterial blood pressure, serum potassium, and plasma renin activity.

Cunningham SK, Moore A, McKenna TJ: Normal cortisol response to corticotropin in patients with secondary adrenal failure. Arch Intern Med 1983; *143*:2276–2279.

Hjortrup A, Kehlet H, Lindholm J, et al.: Value of the 30-minute adrenocorticotropin (ACTH) test in demonstrating hypothalamic-pituitary-adrenocortical insufficiency after acute ACTH deprivation. J Clin Endocrinol Metab 1983; *57*:668–670.

Landon J, Wynn V, James VHT: The adrenocortical response to insulin-induced hypoglycemia. J Endocrinol 1963; *27*:183–192.

Manu P, Howland T: Best conditions for the rapid 1-24-corticotropin stimulation of adrenocortical function. Clin Chem 1983; *29*:1450–1451.

May ME, Carey RM: Rapid adrenocorticotropic hormone test in practice: retrospective review. Am J Med 1985; *79*:679–684.

Spark RF: Simplified assessment of pituitary-adrenal reserve: measurement of serum 11-deoxycortisol and cortisol after metyrapone. Ann Intern Med 1971; *75*:717–720

Tsukada T, Nakai Y, Tsujii S, et al.: Plasma adrenocorticotropin and cortisol responses to ovine corticotropin-releasing factor in patients with adrenocortical insufficiency due to hypothalamic and pituitary disorders. J Clin Endocrinol Metab 1984; *58*:758–761.

CUSHING'S SYNDROME

Background, Pathophysiology

Cushing's syndrome is the result of autonomous, excessive production of cortisol. Normally, secretion of ACTH and cortisol are cyclic; this diurnal rhythm produces highest levels in the early morning and low values in the evening and at night. Most patients with Cushing's syndrome lack the diurnal rhythm; simply maintaining the morning level of cortisol throughout the night leads to the clinical manifestations of Cushing's syndrome.

Chronic cortisol excess causes decreased protein synthesis, nitrogen wasting, glucose intolerance (sometimes with fasting hyperglycemia), and changes in mineral metabolism (sodium retention, wasting of potassium and calcium). While lean body mass is often reduced due to the decrease in protein synthesis, obesity occurs due to increased food intake and depressed turnover of fatty acids. Osteoporosis results from an increase in bone resorption and diminished bone formation. Vertebral compression fractures may occur and cause chronic back pain; the resulting spinal deformity may contribute to the overall appearance of central obesity. Muscle weakness results from diminished muscle protein and possibly from hypokalemia. Thromboembolic disorders are seen due to increases in clotting factors II, V, and VIII. Compromise of the immune system predisposes to opportunistic infections. Secretion of LH is inhibited by excessive cortisol, resulting in menstrual irregularity in females and diminished libido and infertility in males. Emotional disturbances, particularly depression, are common in Cushing's syndrome and sometimes reach psychotic proportions; the mechanism is unknown.

In addition to the excess of cortisol, other adrenal hormones may be produced in excess in Cushing's syndrome. Modest increases in adrenal androgen production are common in pituitary-dependent Cushing's syndrome and lead to hirsutism and acne. Increases in mineralocorticoids (or the mineralocorticoid effect of high levels of cortisol) may be striking in ectopic ACTH production, resulting in hypertension, hypokalemia, and metabolic alkalosis. Adrenal tumors tend to produce an isolated class of steroids; some produce only cortisol, some produce androgens alone, and some only secrete mineralocorticoids (primary aldosteronism). Adrenal carcinomas may also produce estrogens and cause feminization or produce biologically inactive steroids such as 11-deoxycortisol.

The onset and progression of Cushing's syndrome may be gradual or fulminant. Mortality from untreated pituitary-dependent Cushing's syndrome approaches 50% at 5 years. Morbidity and mortality result from diabetes and hypertension-associated vascular complications, osteoporosis with compression fractures, infection, thromboembolic phenomena, and emotional disturbances.

Pituitary-dependent Cushing's syndrome affects females nine times more commonly than males; it may occur at any age but is unusual in children. Adrenal tumors do not show a sexual predominance. Adrenal carcinoma is most common in the fourth and fifth decades. Ectopic ACTH syndrome affects males ten times more often than females.

Most patients with pituitary-dependent Cushing's syndrome have a pituitary tumor. These tumors are usually small, often too small to be visualized with radiographic techniques (CT or MR). While there is some evidence to suggest that there is a hypothalamic cause for these tumors, most evidence supports a primary pituitiary abnormality. The tumors are usually basophilic, but may be chromophobic. The cells contain pro-opiomelanocortin (POMC), the large precursor molecule for ACTH which also includes the amino acid sequences for beta lipotropin, alpha MSH, beta endorphin, and met-enkephalin. Immunoperoxidase staining of these tumors is almost always positive for ACTH, with variable presence of other POMC-derived hormones. ACTH secretion from these tumors is resistant to the inhibitory effect of normal glucocorticoid levels but usually can be suppressed by high doses of glucocorticoids. ACTH response to an intravenous injection of CRH is exaggerated. Recent studies suggest that diurnal variation of ACTH and cortisol secretion may be preserved in some patients but simply manifest at a much higher cortisol level. Up to 10% of these pituitary tumors are large enough to exert some mass effect, including compromise of visual fields, involvement of cranial nerves, or hypopituitarism.

The adrenal glands of patients with pituitary-dependent Cushing's syndrome usually show bilateral diffuse hyperplasia. In some cases, however, the adrenal hyperplasia is nodular. In these patients, it appears that excessive ACTH production from the pituitary initiates nodular hyperplasia of the adrenal glands, which then become autonomous and may continue to cause hypercortisolism despite removal of the pituitary ACTH source.

Clinical Presentation

Patients with Cushing's syndrome usually experience weight gain and a change in appearance. Other frequent complaints include easy fatigue, muscle weakness (especially in proximal muscle groups), easy bruising, poor wound healing, loss of scalp hair, increased face and body hair in women, and alteration in reproductive function (oligomenorrhea or amenorrhea in women, decreased libido and/or impotence in men). Depression and emotional lability are common. Rarely, hyperpigmentation or weight loss may occur, depending on the underlying cause for Cushing's syndrome (most likely with ectopic ACTH production).

Physical findings of Cushing's syndrome may be subtle or quite striking. Typically, the face is round and plethoric ("moon face") and fat pads are increased in the supraclavicular areas and over the upper thoracic spine ("buffalo hump"). Obesity is generalized in 50% of cases; in the remaining 50%, central obesity stands out in striking contrast to relatively slender extremities. The skin is atrophic, sometimes tissue-paper thin, with broad, purple striae over the flanks, breasts, and lower abdomen. Often, there are ecchymoses and purpura. Scalp hair is usually sparse and fine, but there may be increased hair on the face and trunk; acne is often present. Systemic arterial hypertension is common. Generalized muscle wasting may be present, with pronounced weakness in proximal muscle groups.

101

When Cushing's syndrome is due to ectopic production of ACTH by a malignancy, the usual signs may be overshadowed by the cachexia of the underlying malignancy. Hyperpigmentation of the skin and mucous membranes may be seen with the ectopic ACTH syndrome, and less commonly, with pituitary ACTH excess.

Malignant tumors that produce ACTH are usually clinically obvious. The most common malignant tumors associated with *ectopic ACTH* are oat cell carcinoma of the lung, thymoma, carcinoid tumors, and medullary thyroid carcinoma. Patients with ectopic ACTH often lack the obesity and striae that are typical for other forms of Cushing's syndrome, and have instead weight loss, severe hypertension, hypokalemia, myopathy, diabetes, and hyperpigmentation. Their course is often rapidly fatal. Benign tumors (e.g., bronchial carcinoid) that cause ectopic ACTH syndrome may mimic pituitary-dependent Cushing's syndrome on clinical grounds and must be differentiated based on biochemical criteria (Table 6–1) or selective venous sampling for ACTH determination.

Patients with Cushing's syndrome due to a *benign adrenal tumor* are usually found early, at a time when the adrenal lesion is small, because of the clinical manifestations of cortisol excess. In contrast, patients with *adrenal carcinoma* have large bulky tumors, often with local invasion or metastases at the time of presentation. These tumors tend to spread early to liver, lungs, and lymph nodes.

Diagnosis of Cushing's Syndrome

Cushing's syndrome is an uncommon disorder, but the usual signs and symptoms of Cushing's syndrome (e.g., central obesity, hypertension, glucose intolerance, weakness, depression)

Table 6–1. Patterns of Test Results in Cushing's Syndrome

Test	Pituitary Cushing's	Adrenal Tumor	Ectopic ACTH
Plasma ACTH	Normal or high	Low	Very high
Provocative test response*	Yes	No	No
Adrenal CT	Normal or bilateral enlargement	Tumor	Normal or bilateral enlargement

*High-dose dexamethasone, metyrapone, corticotropin-releasing hormone.
(From Watts NB: Cushing's syndrome, *in* Hurst JW (ed): Medicine for the Practicing Physician, 2nd ed. Stoneham MA, Butterworths, 1988. Used with permission.)

are common and nonspecific, frequently being seen in patients without adrenal disease. The diagnosis of Cushing's syndrome should be considered when several of the usual signs and symptoms occur together in the same patient.

The *initial diagnosis* of Cushing's syndrome rests on laboratory evidence of excessive and autonomous cortisol production: increased free cortisol in a 24-hour urine or lack of normal pituitary-adrenal suppression. Occasional patients with Cushing's syndrome do not show these laboratory abnormalities for a variety of reasons; it may be necessary to pursue the investigation further if the clinical suspicion of Cushing's syndrome is strong.

Two simple test strategies are useful in the initial evaluation of Cushing's syndrome. One is measurement of 24-hour *urine free cortisol* ("free" cortisol means that which is freely filtered by the kidney, non-protein bound, and not conjugated to glucuronide or sulfate), which is almost 100% sensitive and specific; false-negative tests are rare, and except when stress leads to an increased cortisol excretion, or in chronic alcoholism, false-positive urine free cortisol levels are seldom seen. Appropriate reference ranges for urine free cortisol should be established by each laboratory; in general, 24-hour urine cortisol <100 μg/24 h would exclude the diagnosis of Cushing's syndrome and levels >150 μg/24 h strongly suggest the diagnosis. Another satisfactory approach is the *overnight dexamethasone suppression test* (protocol p. 210), where 1.0 mg of dexamethasone (a potent glucocorticoid) is given orally at 22:00 h (10:00 PM) and plasma cortisol is measured at 08:00 the next day. With this test, plasma cortisol will be >10 μg/dL in patients with Cushing's syndrome and <5 μg/dL (typically 1 to 2 μg/dL) in most normal subjects. False-positive results are seen more commonly with the overnight dexamethasone suppression test than with urinary free cortisol, and may be due to stress (which overrides the negative feedback of dexamethasone), anticonvulsants (which accelerate the metabolism of dexamethasone), estrogens (which increase cortisol binding globulin), and unipolar depression (which alters the hypothalamic-pituitary-adrenal axis). If a single test is to be done to "rule-out" Cushing's syndrome, urine free cortisol is preferred when a 24-hour urine sample can be obtained, and the overnight dexamethasone suppression test when blood sampling is more convenient.

Other approaches to the initial diagnosis of Cushing's syndrome are fraught with difficulty and are not recommended.

These include measurement of plasma cortisol on AM and PM blood samples to see if a normal diurnal fall in plasma cortisol occurs and determination of 24-hour urine 17-hydroxycorticosteroids (known as 17-OHCS or 17-OHS). These strategies lack sensitivity (i.e., many patients with Cushing's syndrome may have normal results) and specificity (i.e., many patients without Cushing's syndrome will have abnormal results).

In rare patients with Cushing's syndrome, hypercortisolism is mild or intermittent; establishing the diagnosis can be quite difficult when the disorder is strongly suspected on clinical grounds but laboratory tests are normal or equivocal. Conversely, it may be difficult to disprove the diagnosis when the laboratory tests are abnormal but clinical suspicion is low. The classic low dose dexamethasone suppression test (protocol p. 209) described by Liddle (Liddle GW: Tests of pituitary-adrenal suppressibility in the diagnosis of Cushing's syndrome, J Clin Endocrinol Metab 1960; *20*:1539–1560) will usually resolve this question, though rare patients with Cushing's syndrome will show a normal response. Twenty four-hour urine 17-OHCS are measured daily for 2 baseline days and for 2 days with the patient taking dexamethasone 0.5 mg orally every 6 hours. Normal persons show a fall of urinary 17-OHCS to <4.0 mg/g of creatinine. An alternate approach, though less well established, is to measure plasma cortisol at 16:00 on day 2 of low-dose dexamethasone; normal suppression is plasma cortisol <5 μg/dL.

Differential Diagnosis. Once the diagnosis of Cushing's syndrome has been confirmed (elevated urine free cortisol, abnormal overnight or low dose dexamethasone suppression test), additional studies are necessary to establish the etiology. Cushing's syndrome is frequently due to exogenous steroid use; this is usually (but not always) apparent on history. The endogenous disorders that cause Cushing's syndrome may be classified in two ways. The traditional classification includes three general categories: (1) pituitary-dependent Cushing's syndrome (excessive production of ACTH, usually by a pituitary microadenoma) (60 to 70% of cases), (2) adrenal tumors, benign or malignant (25 to 30% of cases), and (3) ectopic production of ACTH (5 to 10% of cases) or corticotropin-releasing hormone (CRH) (rare). A more useful classification is shown in Table 6–2: ACTH-dependent (pituitary or ectopic) and ACTH-independent Cushing's syndrome (adrenal tumors).

Since treatment of Cushing's syndrome usually involves a major surgical procedure, it is desirable to have a high degree

Table 6–2. Causes of Naturally Occurring Cushing's Syndrome

ACTH-Dependent	ACTH-Independent
Pituitary tumor secreting ACTH	Adrenal adenoma
	Adrenal carcinoma
Ectopic production of ACTH	
Ectopic production of CRH	

of certainty regarding the etiology. This usually requires a comprehensive study of each patient; no single test can be relied on in all cases. Unless initial data clearly indicate a particular cause, it is advisable to proceed with complete testing. In several of our cases, analysis of the final test results established a different etiology than the first results suggested.

Plasma ACTH measurement (Fig. 6–3) and adrenal CT scanning should be the initial steps in the differential diagnosis of Cushing's syndrome; the results will allow direction of additional tests toward ACTH-dependent or -independent causes. ACTH-independent Cushing's syndrome patients (adrenal tumor) will have undetectable ACTH levels and unilateral adrenal enlargement. If further confirmation of a unilateral adrenal source is needed, adrenal vein catheterization to demonstrate a cortisol gradient and/or iodocholesterol scanning can be done. If ACTH is elevated and bilateral adrenal enlargement is seen on CT scan, biochemical tests will generally show a pattern that indicates the source of Cushing's syndrome (Table 6–1). The degree of plasma ACTH elevation is useful, being markedly elevated in ectopic ACTH and only slightly increased or "normal" (inappropriately high for the elevated cortisol) in pituitary-dependent Cushing's syndrome (Fig. 6–3). Suppression and stimulation studies usually elicit a response in patients with pituitary-dependent Cushing's syndrome but not in patients with other forms. The classic suppression test is the high-dose dexamethasone test of Liddle (protocol p. 209), 2 mg dexamethasone every 6 hours for 48 hours, response being a decrease of urine 17-OHCS to <50% of baseline, which may be simplified by measuring plasma cortisol the afternoon of the second day (suppression being plasma cortisol <10 µg/dL). Metyrapone, 750 mg every 4 hours for 48 hours normally stimulates ACTH release, the response in patients with pituitary dependent Cushing's syndrome being an increase of urine 17-OHCS to more than three times the baseline. Anomalous results may occur due to episodic or cyclic steroid excess or if the metabolic clearance of dexamethasone is accelerated or prolonged.

CT or MRI of the pituitary should be performed if pituitary-

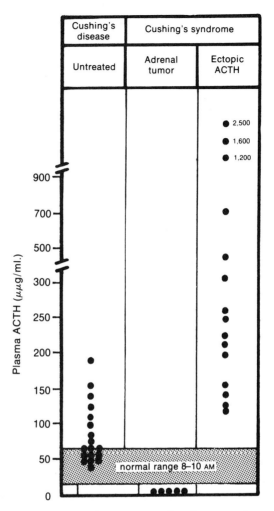

Fig. 6–3. ACTH levels in different causes of Cushing's syndrome. (Adapted from Besser GM: Brit Med J 1968; 4:522, used with permission.)

dependent Cushing's syndrome is suspected, but the pituitary tumors that cause Cushing's syndrome are usually small, often <5 mm in diameter, and can only be demonstrated radiographically in approximately 25% of cases. Routine chest x-rays should be done, with CT scans of the chest reserved for patients suspected of having ectopic ACTH production. Selective venous sampling for ACTH is useful to locate an ectopic vs a pituitary source, and, if pituitary ACTH excess is present, to identify the side of the tumor; the latter is done by bilateral simultaneous catheterization of the inferior petrosal venous sinuses which drain blood from the pituitary gland. ACTH gradients from these tumors are even more pronounced after CRH stimulation. CRH testing may ultimately replace most of the other laboratory studies used for differential diagnosis of Cushing's syndrome; preliminary results indicate an exaggerated ACTH response to CRH in pituitary-dependent Cushing's syndrome, a high baseline and no response in ectopic ACTH, and a low baseline with no response with adrenal tumors.

Treatment of Cushing's Syndrome

Ideal treatment for Cushing's syndrome would (1) correct the hypercortisolism by eliminating the underlying cause, (2) restore normal function of the hypothalamic-pituitary-adrenal axis, and (3) preserve other endocrine functions. These goals are often not fully met by current therapeutic modalities, which for pituitary-dependent Cushing's syndrome (Cushing's disease) include pituitary surgery, bilateral adrenalectomy, pituitary irradiation, drugs that reduce pituitary ACTH release, and drugs that inhibit adrenal hormone synthesis.

Currently, transsphenoidal pituitary surgery is considered the treatment of choice for most patients with pituitary-dependent Cushing's syndrome. A few patients have macroadenomas (≤1 cm in diameter); cure rates for these patients are not as good as when a pituitary microadenoma (<1 cm in diameter) can be identified and selectively removed, resulting in a cure in approximately 85% of cases. If preoperative petrosal vein ACTH samples have shown a gradient of ACTH from one side and a tumor cannot be seen at surgery, a hemihypophysectomy may be done. If a microadenoma still cannot be found, total hypophysectomy is advisable and usually corrects the hypercortisolism, but at the expense of hypopituitarism and the need for life-long replacement therapy. Since the prolonged hypercortisolism of Cushing's disease suppresses the normal hypothalamic-pituitary-adrenal axis, steroid coverage is required during surgery and often for some months after selective tumor removal; some patients must continue steroid treatment lifelong. Pituitary function is usually preserved when selective tumor removal is done. Morbidity (<10%) and mortality (<1%) are acceptably low.

Medical treatment is not recommended as primary therapy for Cushing's syndrome, but may be useful when surgical treatment has failed or is contraindicated, or as an adjunct to other forms of treatment (given preoperatively to improve the patient's state for surgery, or combined with pituitary irradiation to hasten clinical improvement). There are three main classes of drugs to consider: (1) adrenolytic (mitotane, also known as o,p'-DDD), (2) blockers of adrenal steroid synthesis (metyrapone, aminogluthethimide, ketoconazole, and others), and (3) drugs that act on the pituitary or hypothalamus (cyproheptadine), With the exception of ketoconazole, which has proved to be effective and well tolerated, drugs in the first two classes are of limited usefulness because of toxicity.

Cyproheptadine, a serotonin antagonist, has been reported to correct all the abnormalities of Cushing's syndrome in some patients with pituitary-dependent Cushing's syndrome, presumably by reducing a stimulatory effect on the pituitary; response to cyproheptadine suggests that some cases of "pituitary" Cushing's are due to a hypothalamic disorder rather than a primary defect in the pituitary. However, most patients with pituitary-dependent Cushing's syndrome do not respond to this agent, and those who do are often bothered by side effects such as severe lethargy or excessive appetite.

Bilateral adrenalectomy is a more traumatic operation than transsphenoidal pituitary surgery and is frequently complicated by wound infection, poor healing, and thromboembolic complications. Morbidity occurs in 15 to 20% of patients, and mortality in 2 to 5%. While adrenalectomy corrects the hypercortisolism of pituitary-dependent Cushing's syndrome (unless an extra-adrenal remnant is left behind), patients so treated depend on lifelong glucocorticoid and mineralocorticoid replacement. Up to 30% of patients treated by adrenalectomy will develop Nelson's syndrome, an aggressive ACTH-secreting tumor that does not respond well to treatment.

Conventional pituitary irradiation (4500 to 5000 rads) is effective in correcting hypercortisolism in 20 to 40% of patients with pituitary-dependent Cushing's syndrome and leads to some improvement in another 40%. However, irradiation may cause deficiencies of other pituitary hormones and rarely, optic nerve damage, brain necrosis, or cranial neoplasms. Clinical improvement after irradiation may not be apparent for 1 to 2 years after treatment. Proton beam irradiation is limited to two centers in the U.S. because it requires specialized equipment; it gives a higher percentage of "cures" than conventional radiation, up to 90 to 95%, and has a more rapid onset of effect, but results in a higher frequency of hypopituitarism. Proton beam irradiation cannot be used for tumors with extrasellar extension.

Treatment of choice for adrenal tumors causing Cushing's syndrome is tumor removal. The contralateral adrenal should eventually regain normal function, though steroid replacement may be needed for 6 to 12 months, until the hypothalamic-pituitary axis has recovered. For adrenal carcinoma with metastases, debulking the tumor mass surgically is advisable. The adrenolytic agent mitotane usually reduces cortisol production and helps control the signs and symptoms of Cushing's syndrome; it may also cause some reduction of tumor size, and in a few cases, apparent "cures." Radiation and other cancer chemotherapeutic drugs have not proved effective.

In Cushing's syndrome due to ectopic production of ACTH, treatment should be directed at the underlying tumor. If signs or symptoms of hypercortisolism are severe, ketoconazole or another inhibitor of adrenal hormone synthesis can be useful.

Aron DC, Tyrrell JB, Fitzgerald PA, et al.: Cushing's syndrome: problems in diagnosis. Medicine 1983; 60:25–35.

Chrousos GP, Schuermeyer TH, Doppman J, et al.: Clinical applications of corticotropin releasing factor. Ann Intern Med 1985; 102:344–358.

Dunlap NE, Grizzle WE, Siegel AL: Cushing's syndrome: screening methods in hospitalized patients. Arch Path Lab Med 1985; 109:222–229.

Gold EM: The Cushing syndromes: changing views of diagnosis and treatment. Ann Intern Med 1979; 90:829–844.

Ross EJ, Marshall-Jones P, Friedman M: Cushing's syndrome: diagnostic criteria. Quart J Med 1966; 59:149–192.

CONGENITAL ADRENAL HYPERPLASIA

Background, Pathophysiology

Congenital adrenal hyperplasia is also known as "adrenogenital syndrome" because of the striking genital abnormalities seen in affected infants. One of several enzyme deficiencies may be the cause. All of these disorders are transmitted by autosomal recessive inheritance. Table 6–3 shows the various types of defects included under the heading congenital adrenal hyperplasia and Figure 6–4 shows the synthetic pathways and enzymes. The common feature of these disorders is a diminished capacity for cortisol production, which results in excessive production of ACTH by the pituitary gland, in turn causing hyperplasia of the adrenal glands and overproduction of precursor steroids. Some of these precursors have biologic activity and some are shunted to other pathways (e.g., from the glucocorticoid pathway to the androgen pathway). Depending on

Table 6–3. Types of Congenital Adrenal Hyperplasia

Deficient Enzyme	Immediate Precursors	Deficiencies	Excesses
21-Hydroxylase	17-OH Progesterone Progesterone	G M	A
11-Hydroxylase	11-Deoxycortisol	G M (aldosterone)	M (DOC) A
3-β-Hydroxysteroid dehydrogenase*	Pregnenolone 17-OH Pregnenolone DHEA	G M GS	Weak androgens (DHEA)
17-Hydroxylase	Progesterone Pregnenolone DOC	G GS	M (aldosterone)
20,22 Desmolase*	Cholesterol	G, M, GS	None

*Also affects gonads

Abbreviations: A, androgens; G, glucocorticoids; M, mineralocorticoids; GS, gonadal steroids (testosterone and estrogen); DOC, deoxycorticosterone; DHEA, dehydroepiandrosterone

(From Watts NB: Congenital adrenal hyperplasia, *in* Hurst JW (ed): Medicine for the Practicing Physician, 2nd ed. Stoneham MA, Butterworths, 1988.)

the specific enzyme that is deficient, there may also be insufficient production of mineralocorticoids, adrenal androgens, or gonadal steroids (testosterone and estrogens). Biologically active precursors that may accumulate include androgens and mineralocorticoids. Clinical manifestations vary depending on hormone classes that are deficient, those that are excessive, and the degree of completeness of the enzyme deficiency.

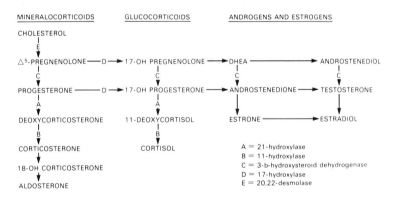

Fig. 6–4. Pathways of adrenal hormone synthesis. (From Watts NB: Congenital adrenal hyperplasia, *in* Hurst JW (ed): Medicine for the Practicing Physician, 2nd ed. Stoneham MA, Butterworths, 1988.

21-hydroxylase deficiency is by far the most common form of congenital adrenal hyperplasia, occurring in 1/10,000 Caucasian births. In affected kindreds, HLA typing is useful for detection of heterozygote carriers and for prenatal diagnosis (the gene for this disorder is closely linked to HLA genes, is more frequent with Bw47, Aw33, and B14 and less frequent with B8). 21-Hydroxylase is necessary for conversion of 17-hydroxyprogesterone to 11-deoxycortisol and on to cortisol, and of progesterone to deoxycorticosterone and on to aldosterone (Fig. 6–4). The result of a complete 21-hydroxylase deficiency is a rise in all compounds in the steroidogenic pathways that precede this enzymatic step–progesterone, 17-hydroxyprogesterone, and adrenal androgens (mainly androstenedione, which is converted to testosterone in peripheral tissues). Urinary excretion of 17-ketosteroids is increased, as is that of pregnanetriol, the most important metabolite of 17-hydroxyprogesterone.

In the most severe form of 21-hydroxylase deficiency, a salt-wasting crisis generally occurs 6 to 14 days after birth, manifest by severe dehydration, hyponatremia, hyperkalemia, acidosis, and shock. In the incomplete form, salt wasting is mild or does not occur. In both types, affected female infants have ambiguous external genitalia, sometimes even a male appearance when the defect is severe, though internal genitalia (uterus, tubes, and ovaries) are usually normal; in milder cases, the patient may appear normal at birth, with signs of virilization beginning at age 3 or so. Affected males do not usually show any genital abnormalities at birth, but begin to show signs of puberty, such as growth of pubic hair and enlargement of the penis (but not the testes) within a few years. Both males and females show rapid early growth, but final height is reduced due to premature closure of the epiphyses.

21-Hydroxylase deficiency may become apparent at puberty, where it is termed "late onset," "attenuated," or "acquired." The term "acquired" is a misnomer, since the enzyme deficiency is present at birth. At the time of puberty, affected females show signs of hirsutism and oligomenorrhea similar to the polycystic ovary syndrome. Basal serum concentrations of 17-hydroxyprogesterone are elevated in some women with this condition, but not all. An exaggerated rise of serum 17-hydroxyprogesterone after ACTH stimulation (60 minutes after 250 μg cosyntropin IV, serum 17-hydroxyprogesterone <900 ng/dL in normals, >2000 ng/dL in the late-onset form, and >16,000 ng/dL in the classic form) serves as a useful diagnostic.

test. However, some women with the biochemical abnormalities do not develop hirsutism, indicating that end-organ sensitivity plays a definite role in the phenotypic expression. Since "late-onset" congenital adrenal hyperplasia does not appear to be a common cause of hirsutism, routine screening of hirsute women for 21-hydroxylase deficiency is not warranted.

11-Hydroxylase deficiency occurs in about 1/200,000 live births in this country. This enzyme promotes the conversion of 11-deoxycortisol to cortisol and the conversion of deoxycorticosterone down the pathway to aldosterone. Deoxycorticosterone accumulates and exerts sufficient mineralocorticoid activity to cause retention of sodium and water, arterial hypertension, and suppression of plasma renin activity; however, hypertension may not present until adulthood. Hypokalemia is uncommon in these patients. Androgen excess leads to female pseudohermaphroditism at birth and postnatal virilization in both males and females. Mildly affected males may present only with hypertension or gynecomastia (from conversion of androgens to estrogens).

3-β-Hydroxysteroid dehydrogenase deficiency is rare. The inheritance is autosomal recessive. A complete deficiency of this enzyme is incompatible with life; a partial defect results in deficient synthesis of glucocorticoids, mineralocorticoids, and gonadal steroids. Urinary 17-ketosteroids are increased, as are plasma levels of 17-hydroxypregnenolone and other precursor steroids. Some virilization occurs, probably from conversion of DHEA to testosterone in the liver, where the enzyme seems to be under separate genetic control. Males show varying degrees of pseudohermaphroditism. Salt wasting may be present. In females, there is often slight clitoral enlargement; virilization may appear in childhood or adolescence.

In *17-hydroxylase deficiency,* further conversion of progesterone and pregnenolone to cortisol or adrenal androgens is impaired and production of gonadal steroids is reduced. There is excessive production of deoxycorticosterone, a strong mineralocorticoid which suppresses plasma renin activity and aldosterone production. Affected subjects show hypertension and hypokalemic alkalosis. 17-Ketosteroid excretion is low. In females, there is sexual infantilism and in males, varying degrees of pseudohermaphroditism. Pubic and axillary hair is scant. Patients may present as phenotypic females with primary amenorrhea and hypertension.

20,22-Desmolase deficiency is rare. This enzyme is important quite early in steroid synthesis, and a complete deficiency is incompatible with life. Even with replacement therapy, all affected infants have died.

Severely affected infants with congenital adrenal hyperplasia will die if the disorder is not compensated or treated. Females with a defect that is mild or occurs late will experience short stature, virilization, menstrual irregularities, and infertility. Males have short stature and are usually infertile. With early diagnosis and proper management, these patients can lead a perfectly normal life in terms of sexual development and fertility; final stature is often somewhat decreased because of difficulty in optimizing glucocorticoid therapy.

Clinical Presentation

Clinical manifestations of congenital adrenal hyperplasia vary, and include (in different combinations, depending on the defect) abnormal external genitalia in newborns of both sexes (with females sometimes appearing as "cryptorchid" males), salt-wasting crisis in neonates, rapid early growth but eventual short stature in both sexes, early sexual maturation in males, hirsutism or virilization in females (often beginning in childhood but sometimes presenting at adolescence), and in the rare varieties, failure to undergo puberty, and hypertension with hypokalemia.

The signs and symptoms of the different varieties of congenital adrenal hyperplasia vary with the specific enzyme that is deficient and with the completeness of the defect. Table 6–3 lists the enzyme abnormalities, the specific steroid compounds that are produced in excess, and the classes of adrenal hormones that are deficient or excessive.

Symptoms of congential adrenal hyperplasia include those related to:

1. *mineralocorticoid deficiency*—anorexia, nausea, vomiting, dehydration, and circulatory collapse
2. *androgen excess*—rapid early growth in both sexes, increased body and facial hair in females and early sexual development in males, infertility in both sexes
3. *gonadal hormone deficiency (testosterone and estrogens)*—failure of puberty to occur

Abnormal physical findings can be explained by the types of steroid compounds that are deficient or increased and the severity of the enzyme defect. These include:

1. *in-utero androgen excess*—female pseudohermaphroditism, with genital abnormalities ranging from severe (the

113

appearance of a cryptorchid male) to moderate (labioscrotal fusion, hypospadias, clitoromegaly) to mild (slight clitoral enlargement); no manifestations in males

2. *postnatal androgen excess*—both males and females show an early rapid growth in height; however, excessive androgens lead to premature closure of the epiphyses and a reduced final stature, males show signs of sexual maturation beginning at age 3 or 4 (pubic hair growth and enlargement of the penis, but the testes remain small); in females, continued androgen excess is manifest by signs of virilization such as increased face and body hair, oily skin, acne, deepening of the voice, and a male body habitus; menses may be irregular

3. *intrauterine androgen deficiency*—males show incomplete development of male external genital structures, including a bifid scrotum, micropenis, and varying degrees of hypospadias; no effect in females

4. *deficient gonadal steroid production* (testosterone and estrogens)—failure to undergo puberty or develop secondary sex characteristics

5. *mineralocorticoid deficiency*—hypotension, dehydration, and shock (salt-wasting crisis), usually manifest in the first few weeks after birth

6. *mineralocorticoid excess*—fluid retention and hypertension

7. *severe ACTH excess*—hyperpigmentation of the skin and mucous membranes

Diagnosis of Congenital Adrenal Hyperplasia

The diagnosis of congenital adrenal hyperplasia is made by demonstrating an excessive amount of the specific precursor steroids in blood or urine (Table 6–4), then showing that these compounds can be suppressed by administration of glucocorticoids. In all varieties (except for 17-hydroxylase deficiency, which is rare), urinary 17-ketosteroid excretion is increased. Specific precursors of cortisol can be measured in plasma: 17-hydroxyprogesterone in 21-hydroxylase deficiency; 11-deoxycortisol in 11-hydroxylase deficiency; 17-hydroxypregnenolone in 3-β-steroid dehydrogenase deficiency. In classic cases, basal concentrations of these steroids are sufficiently elevated to establish the diagnosis. In mild cases or heterozygotes, it may be necessary to measure the steroids after stimulation with ACTH to show the abnormality. (New MI, Lorenzen F, Lerner AJ et al.:

Table 6–4. Hormone Reference Data for Diagnosis of Congenital Adrenal Hyperplasia*

Compound	Age	Normal Range
URINE		
17-Ketosteroids	2 weeks–2 years	0–1 mg/day
	2–6 years	0–2
	6–10 years	1–4
	10–12 years	1–6
	12–14	3–10
	14–16	5–12
	male adult	9–22
	female adult	6–15
Pregnanetriol	2 weeks–2 years	0.02–0.2 mg/day
	2–5 years	<0.5
	5–15 years	<1.5
	adult	<2.0
PLASMA		
Androstenedione	males 1–3 months	20–45 ng/dL
	3–5 months	10–40
	adult	75–125
	female 1–3 months	15–25
	3–5 months	10–15
	adult	110–190
Dehydroepiandrosterone	child	1–3 ng/mL
	male adult	1.7–4.2
	female adult	2.0–5.2
Deoxycorticosterone	adult	40–150 pg/mL (approx)
11-Deoxycortisol	adult	0.5–1.2 μg/dL
17-Hydroxypregnenolone	adult	0.3–3.5 ng/mL
17-Hydroxyprogesterone	male (child)	0.1–0.3 ng/mL
	male (adult)	0.2–1.8
	female (child)	0.2–0.5
	female (follicular)	0.2–0.8
	female (luteal)	0.8–3.0
	post ACTH stim.	<3.3†

*Reference ranges for plasma aldosterone, estradiol, and testosterone should be readily available from most commercial laboratories

†See New MI, Lorenzen F, Lerner AJ, et al: J Clin Endocrinol Metab 1983; 57:320–326.

(From Watts NB: Congenital adrenal hyperplasia, in Hurst JW (ed): Medicine for the Practicing Physician, 2nd ed. Stoneham MA, Butterworths, 1988.)

Genotyping steroid 21-hydroxylase deficiency: Hormonal reference data. J Clin Endocrinol Metab 1983; 57:320–326) have developed a useful nomogram for basal and ACTH-stimulated 17-hydroxyprogesterone measurements in 21-hydroxylase deficiency (Fig. 6–5). If increased values are found, congenital adrenal hyperplasia can be distinguished from hormone-pro-

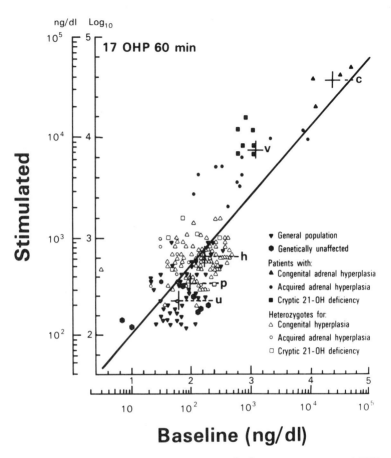

Fig. 6–5. Nomogram relating basal serum 17-hydroxyprogesterone to ACTH-stimulated values in normal individuals and subjects with congenital adrenal hyperplasia due to 21-hydroxylase deficiency (From White et al.: N Engl J Med 1987; *316*:1519; figure copyright Maria I. New, M.D., 1982, used with permission.)

ducing neoplasms by demonstrating correction of the hormone elevation with glucocorticoid treatment; this often can be accomplished simply by instituting treatment with hydrocortisone and repeating the abnormal tests after 3 or 4 weeks, or as a standard low dose dexamethasone suppression test (see Cushing's syndrome, p. 209). Prenatal diagnosis can sometimes be made by hormone measurement in amniotic fluid, and, in the case of 21-hydroxylase deficiency, HLA typing. HLA typing is also useful to identify heterozygote carriers of 21-hydroxylase deficiency.

When the clinical presentation is an infant with ambiguous

genitalia, karyotype analysis must be done to rule out sex chromosome abnormalities. Other considerations in patients with similar manifestations include intrauterine androgen exposure, partial androgen resistance, 5-α-reductase deficiency, or developmental genital abnormalities such as hypospadias and cryptorchidism. Demonstration of abnormal steroid production establishes the diagnosis of congenital adrenal hyperplasia, though levels may not be diagnostically increased until 2 to 3 weeks after birth.

The presentation of congenital adrenal hyperplasia may be delayed until childhood. Females with virilization must be evaluated for androgen-producing tumors of the ovaries or adrenals, and males showing early signs of sexual maturation must be tested for CNS tumors and other causes of early pubertal development.

In adolescent females, late-onset congenital hyperplasia must be differentiated from virilizing adrenal or ovarian tumors, idiopathic hirsutism, and polycystic ovary syndrome. Measurement of blood levels of testosterone and DHEAS before and after dexamethasone are useful, as are CT scans of the adrenals and ultrasound of the ovaries.

Treatment of Congenital Adrenal Hyperplasia

Lifelong glucocorticoid replacement is essential in all cases of congenital adrenal hyperplasia. Glucocorticoids restore normal feedback inhibition to the pituitary gland, resulting in diminished ACTH secretion and reduced stimulation of the adrenal glands to make the undesirable steroid precursors. In infants, the usual regimen is cortisone acetate 12.5 mg/M^2/day given as an IM injection of three times the daily dose every 3 days. After 2 years of age, the oral route is preferred; because oral activity of cortisone acetate or hydrocortisone is less than parenteral, the usual oral dose of cortisone acetate is 25 mg/M^2/day (equivalent to hydrocortisone 20 mg/M^2/day). For adults, a typical schedule is hydrocortisone 10 mg three times a day. This differs from the recommended schedule for adrenal insufficiency patients, where the usual dose is 20 mg in the morning and 10 mg in the afternoon; in congenital adrenal hyperplasia, including an evening dose helps dampen the expected early morning surge of ACTH. Glucocorticoid therapy must be monitored closely in these patients and the dose adjusted to meet individual needs. Excessive doses lead to growth retardation and features of Cushing's syndrome, while an insufficient dose will not suppress the undesired steroids. Growth rate, bone age, and steroid hormone production (either urine 17-ketosteroids or plasma levels of steroid precursors) should be checked at regular intervals.

Mineralocorticoid replacement may not be needed if salt wasting is mild, where simply increasing dietary sodium may be sufficient. Medication, when required, is usually provided as fludrocortisone (Florinef), usual adult dose range is 0.05 to 0.2 mg daily, and in infants, deoxycorticosterone acetate (Percorten), which can be given by IM injection (usual dose 1 to 2 mg daily) or as subcutaneous pellets. The salt-losing tendency may decrease by age 5 or so, allowing mineralocorticoid treatment to be reduced or discontinued. For *mineralocorticoid excess,* spironolactone (Aldactone), an inhibitor of aldosterone, is usually sufficient in a dose of 25 mg four times a day. Mineralocorticoid therapy can be monitored by measuring blood pressure, serum electrolytes, and, if necessary, plasma renin activity; spironolactone therapy can be assessed by following these same parameters. In cases in which gonadal steroid production is deficient, it is necessary to institute estrogen or testosterone replacement at the time of puberty.

Surgical correction of the genital abnormalities in females is usually quite successful. Division of the fused labia and recession (*not* resection) of the clitoris should be done in the first year of life; vaginal plastic surgery is probably best deferred until puberty. If male genital deformities are mild, surgery can be done to repair scrotal and penile abnormalities. However, surgery is not always satisfactory in chromosomal males with intrauterine androgen deficiency and incomplete development of male external genitalia. A decision on gender assignment should be made early; if surgery cannot provide genitalia that will be sufficient for sexual performance as a male, the parents should be encouraged to consider having the gonadal tissue removed and rearing the patient as a female.

Genetic counselling is an important part of management, both for the parents of an affected child, as well as for the patient. All varieties of congenital adrenal hyperplasia are inherited in an autosomal recessive pattern. Heterozygotes can be identified by ACTH testing or, in the case of 21-hydroxylase deficiency, by HLA typing. Parents (and eventually the patient) should be assured that sexual function can be normal despite ambiguities of external genitalia.

Until full skeletal growth is complete, children with congenital adrenal hyperplasia should be seen frequently, about every 3 months. Linear growth and weight gain should be carefully plotted, periodic x-ray studies for bone age performed, and urine or blood steroid measurements done to assess the adequacy of suppressive therapy. Most authorities favor measurement of urinary 17-ketosteroids, with normal values being the best indication of adequate suppression. In patients with mineralocorticoid abnormalities, blood pressure and serum electrolytes should be monitored as well. Once growth and development are complete, visits once or twice a year should be adequate.

(Editorial): Congenital adrenal hyperplasia. Lancet 1987; 2:663–664.

Bongiovanni AM: Acquired adrenal hyperplasia with special reference to 3-β-hydroxysteroid dehydrogenase. Fertil Steril 1981; 35:599–608.

Brodie BL, Wentz AC: Late onset congenital adrenal hyperplasia: a gynecologist's perspective. Fertil Steril 1987; 48:175–188.

Chetkowski RJ, DeFazio J, Shamonki I, et al.: The incidence of late-onset congenital hyperplasia due to 21-hydroxylase deficiency among hirsute women. J Clin Endocrinol Metab 1984; 58:595–598.

Kuttenn F, Couillin P, Girard F, et al.: Late-onset adrenal hyperplasia in hirsutism. N Engl J Med 1985; 313:224–231.

Migeon CJ: Diagnosis and management of congenital adrenal hyperplasia. Hosp Practice 1977; 12:75–82.

White PG, New MI, Dupont D: Congenital adrenal hyperplasia. N Engl J Med 1987; 316:1519–1524, 1580–1586.

Zachman M, Tassinari D, Prader A: Clinical and biochemical variability of congenital adrenal hyperplasia due to 11-β-hydroxylase deficiency. A study of 25 patients. J Clin Endocrinol Metab 1983; 56:222–229.

THE INCIDENTALLY DISCOVERED ADRENAL MASS

With the routine application of imaging techniques such as computed tomography, abnormalities of the adrenal glands are being found in 0.5 to 1.0% of asymptomatic patients. What are these masses, and how should they be evaluated?

Primary or secondary neoplasms, hemorrhage, and inflammatory diseases involving one or both adrenal glands may present as an "incidentally" discovered adrenal mass. Many of these are small benign tumors such as myelolipomas. The first step in the evaluation should be to review the patient's history and physical examination. Is there a known malignancy or inflammatory disease that might involve the adrenal (e.g., lung or breast carcinoma, tuberculosis)? Is the patient receiving anticoagulants? Does the patient show any signs of adrenal hormone excess (evidence of Cushing's syndrome, androgen, estrogen, mineralocorticoid, or catecholamine excess)? If the answer is "yes" to any of these questions, specific tests should be done to follow up that possibility. If the answer is "no" on all counts, at least one 24-hour urine determination should be done to evaluate the possibility of a hormone-producing tumor. Urinary metanephrine is the best single test to rule out pheochromocytoma. Adrenal cortical carcinomas may produce inactive or minimally active precursors that would be included in measurements of 17-keto-, 17-ketogenic-, or 17-hydroxysteroids. While magnetic resonance (MR) techniques provide some indication of benign vs malignant tumor, there are too many false-positive and false-negative results to rely on. If there is no clinical or laboratory evidence that the tumor is functioning, the size of the tumor determines the next step. Tumors <3 cm in diameter are unlikely to be malignant, and should simply be restudied by repeat CT scan 6 to 12 months later. Lesions between 3 and 6 cm can be evaluated with relative safety by CT-directed percutaneous needle biopsy. The cytologic diagnosis of benign vs malignant primary adrenal tumors is often not possible, but needle aspiration may permit diagnosis of myelolipoma vs adrenal cortical tumor vs metastatic carcinoma. Lesions >6 cm in diameter should be removed surgically, if the patient's condition permits.

Belldegrun A, Hussain S, Seltzer SE, et al.: Incidentally discovered mass of the adrenal gland. Surg Gynecol Obstet 1986; *163*:203–208.
Copeland PM: The incidentally discovered adrenal mass. Ann Intern Med 1983; *98*:940–945.

ALDOSTERONE, PHEOCHROMOCYTOMA AND CATECHOLAMINES

These topics are discussed in Chapter 7.

7

Adrenal Medulla, Mineralocorticoids, Hypokalemia

ADRENAL MEDULLA, CATECHOLAMINES

Background, Pathophysiology

Three hormones are considered catecholamines: dopamine, norepinephrine, and epinephrine. The pathways for synthesis are shown in Figure 7–1. Dopamine serves primarily as a neurotransmitter in certain areas of the brain and spinal cord (particularly the anterior and posterior hypothalamus). Endocrine effects of dopamine include stimulation of growth hormone and suppression of prolactin. Norepinephrine serves primarily as a neurotransmitter for postganglionic sympathetic nerves. Stimuli for release of norepinephrine include upright posture, exercise, and stress. Patients with norepinephrine deficiency due to autonomic neuropathy may present with postural hypotension.

Two of these catecholamines are secreted by the adrenal medullae and act at distant target sites: norepinephrine and epinephrine. The main clinical disorder related to catecholamines is pheochromocytoma, in which norepinephrine (and sometimes epinephrine) is produced in excess. Both epinephrine and norepinephrine have marked influences on the vascular system; epinephrine also influences metabolic processes, especially carbohydrate metabolism. Epinephrine and norepinephrine produce divergent effects in certain tissues. The existence of two types of adrenergic receptors with different sensitivities for the two catecholamines, alpha and beta, accounts for the varying responses. Alpha receptors interact with both epinephrine and norepinephrine; beta receptors respond to epinephrine but are relatively insensitive to norepinephrine. Table 7–1 lists the different responses expected from these receptors.

After release, norepinephrine is largely subject to reuptake

121

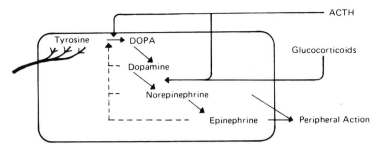

Fig. 7–1. Catecholamine synthesis in the adrenal medulla.

Table 7–1. Physiologic Responses Induced by Alpha and Beta Receptors

Site of Effect	Alpha Response	Beta Response
Vascular beds	Vasoconstriction	Vasodilatation
Intestinal smooth muscle	Relaxation	Relaxation
Bronchial smooth muscle	None	Relaxation
Cardiac contraction	None	Increase
Heart rate	None	Increase
Pupils	Dilatation	None
Piloerection	Stimulation	None
Insulin release	Inhibition	Stimulation
Blood glucose	Increase	Decrease

(From Chattoraj SC and Watts NB: Endocrinology, *in* Tietz NB (ed), Textbook of Endocrinology, 2nd ed. Philadelphia, WB Saunders, 1987, p. 1137.)

by nerve endings and metabolized; only small amounts are excreted unchanged in the urine. Both epinephrine and norepinephrine have short half-lives (a few minutes) in the circulation. Two enzymatic events are responsible for inactivation of catecholamines. Catechol-O-methyl transferase (COMT), present in most tissues (especially in liver, kidney, and erythrocytes), leads to the formation of normetanephrine and metanephrine. These products are partially excreted in the urine but also undergo deamination by monoamine oxidase (MAO) and oxidation to vanillylmandelic acid (VMA), or reduction to methoxyhydroxyphenyl-glycol (MHPG); these end products are subsequently excreted. The final metabolite of dopamine is homovanillic acid (HVA). The degradation pathways for catecholamines are shown in Figure 7–2. Urinary measurements of these metabolites reflect the total production of norepinephrine and epinephrine.

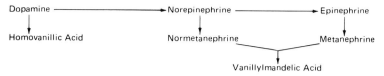

Fig. 7–2. Metabolic degradation pathways of catecholamines.

Clinical Presentation

Manifestations of excess catecholamines include hypertension, weight loss, glucose intolerance, "spells" of palpitations, perspiration, pounding headache, and pallor (the "four p's"), tremor, and nervousness. These signs and symptoms commonly occur in the absence of disease, triggered by stress or anxiety. They may be produced by such endocrine problems as falling blood glucose or hyperthyroidism, or they may result from overproduction of norepinephrine or epinephrine or both by tumors.

Pheochromocytoma is a rare disease, but the signs and symptoms are so striking and cure so rewarding that it receives a great deal of discussion. Patients with pathologic excess of catecholamines typically complain of "spells" as outlined above. In addition, arterial hypertension is common, sustained in many patients and labile or intermittent in some, who often experience a drop in blood pressure on standing. Sometimes the hypertension reaches crisis proportions. Some of these tumors secrete little active catecholamine because of uptake and metabolism by the tumor; patients with this type of tumor may have few if any signs and symptoms of catecholamine excess but have instead a palpable abdominal mass or an incidentally discovered adrenal mass on CT scan.

Benign or malignant neoplasms that produce catecholamines may arise anywhere in the autonomic nervous system or in the adrenal medulla. Tumors of the adrenal medulla are correctly called pheochromocytomas. Those that occur in extra-adrenal sites are termed paragangliomas. The behavior of these tumors fits roughly the "rule of 10": 90% in the adrenal medulla, 10% extra-adrenal; 10% bilateral; 10% malignant; 10% familial or in kindreds with multiple endocrine neoplasia. Malignant tumors and bilateral tumors occur more frequently in children. Hormonally "silent" tumors are more likely to be malignant. The clinical picture of pheochromocytoma rarely is due to adrenal medullary hyperplasia in the absence of tumor.

Who should be tested for pheochromocytoma? These tumors

are rare. Although hypertension is a common sign of pheochromocytoma, this catecholamine-secreting tumor accounts for <0.5% of all cases of hypertension. Screening or testing of all patients with hypertension for pheochromocytoma is not cost effective. However, patients who have labile hypertension, postural hypotension, or symptoms of adrenergic excess should be tested. Pheochromocytomas are familial in about 10% of cases and occur in kindreds with multiple endocrine neoplasia syndromes IIa and IIb. Patients in kindreds known to have multiple endocrine neoplasia syndrome should be considered for testing, even when they are asymptomatic. Also, any patient found to have an adrenal mass or enlargement by CT or MR should be tested. Despite selectivity in testing, false-positive test results are frequent and are much more common than true-positive tests.

Diagnosis of Pheochromocytoma

A number of aspects of normal physiology make it difficult for any single test of catecholamine production or action to be satisfactory for screening or for definitively diagnosing pheochromocytoma. Norepinephrine levels in plasma usually reflect only a small fraction of the concentration of norepinephrine at the nerve ending. The half-life of catecholamines in plasma is brief. Rapid and striking increases in plasma catecholamine concentrations are induced by pain, stress, upright posture, exercise, hypoglycemia, hypovolemia, cold, hypoxia, hypercapnia, or the mental states of anxiety or anger. Also, there is a diurnal variation of catecholamines, with the zenith in the morning and the nadir at night. In addition, medications may change catecholamine concentration. Beta-adrenergic blockers, peripheral alpha-adrenergic blockers (prazocin), vasodilators, and theophylline increase norepinephrine levels; central alpha-adrenergic blockers (clonidine), alpha-methyl dopa, bromocriptine, and phenothiazines decrease the levels of norepinephrine. Other factors that further complicate the clinical application of these tests include drug interference with specific assay procedures and the conditions of sample collection. Furthermore, patients with pheochromocytoma may release catecholamines only intermittently, or the uptake and degradation of catecholamines will result in normal levels of free catecholamines in blood and urine despite striking increases in urinary metabolites, metanephrines and VMA.

Measurement of *urinary metanephrines* (actually, metanephrine plus normetanephrine) is recommended as the initial screening test for pheochromocytoma. This test has almost no false-negatives (nearly 100% sensitivity) in unstressed subjects. Elevations are often seen in times of severe stress, but results are likely to be normal when the test is repeated. A 24-hour urine collection is desirable and provides an "integrated" reflection of catecholamine production. A 12-hour overnight sample can be satisfactory, provided that urinary metanephrine is expressed per gram of creatinine; a normal metanephrine/creatinine ratio is 2.2 μg metanephrine per g creatinine. In patients with intermittent signs and symptoms, a 2-, 4- or 6-hour collection during a "spell" should be done.

If a pheochromocytoma cannot be diagnosed or excluded with urine metanephrine measurement, additional studies are needed. A logical approach is presented in Figure 7–3. Measurement of urinary VMA or catecholamines or both is useful in patients with a low probability of pheochromocytoma but an elevated urinary metanephrine/creatinine ratio, or in subjects with normal urinary metanephrine but who are highly suspect for pheochromocytoma. Urinary VMA and catecholamine determinations are more specific (fewer false-positives) but are less sensitive (more false-negatives) and are more subject to drug interferences than are urinary metanephrine measurements.

Some authorities advocate measurement of *plasma catecholamines* as an initial test for pheochromocytoma; however, it is generally felt that plasma catecholamine measurements should be used only in selected instances, specifically patients with a high suspicion for pheochromocytoma but normal urinary metanephrines. A few patients with pheochromocytoma who have normal levels of catecholamines, metanephrine, and VMA in urine, but definite elevations of norepinephrine or epinephrine in plasma have been reported. Conditions of sampling for plasma catecholamine measurement are highly important. Blood for catecholamine determination should be drawn in the morning after 30 minutes of rest in the recumbent position, ideally from an indwelling needle placed 20 to 30 minutes beforehand (venipuncture may cause stress and increase plasma levels of catecholamines). Plasma must be promptly separated from blood. If measurements of basal levels of catecholamines and metabolites fail to establish or exclude the diagnosis of pheochromocytoma, pharmacologic tests to suppress or stimulate catecholamines may be considered.

The use of agents to stimulate the release of catecholamines has largely been stopped because of the risk of precipitating a

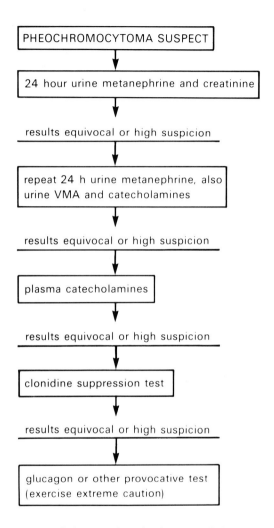

```
┌─────────────────────────────────────────┐
│  PHEOCHROMOCYTOMA SUSPECT                 │
└─────────────────────────────────────────┘
                    │
                    ▼
┌─────────────────────────────────────────┐
│  24 hour urine metanephrine and creatinine│
└─────────────────────────────────────────┘
                    │
                    ▼
    results equivocal or high suspicion
    ─────────────────────────────────────
                    │
                    ▼
┌─────────────────────────────────────────┐
│  repeat 24 h urine metanephrine, also     │
│  urine VMA and catecholamines             │
└─────────────────────────────────────────┘
                    │
                    ▼
    results equivocal or high suspicion
    ─────────────────────────────────────
                    │
                    ▼
┌─────────────────────────────────────────┐
│  plasma catecholamines                    │
└─────────────────────────────────────────┘
                    │
                    ▼
    results equivocal or high suspicion
    ─────────────────────────────────────
                    │
                    ▼
┌─────────────────────────────────────────┐
│  clonidine suppression test               │
└─────────────────────────────────────────┘
                    │
                    ▼
    results equivocal or high suspicion
    ─────────────────────────────────────
                    │
                    ▼
┌─────────────────────────────────────────┐
│  glucagon or other provocative test       │
│  (exercise extreme caution)               │
└─────────────────────────────────────────┘
```

Fig. 7–3. Recommended approach to the diagnosis of pheochromocytoma. If clinical suspicion is low, a normal 24-hour urine metanephrine result is sufficient to rule out the diagnosis. If clinical suspicion is strong and 24-hour urine metanephrine level is clearly elevated (assuming no interfering medication or conditions), localization studies can be done. This complete sequence is needed only for the patient when clinical suspicion is strong and initial studies are normal or equivocal.

hypertensive crisis in patients with pheochromocytoma as well as frequent false-positive and false-negative responses. For patients in whom the diagnosis of pheochromocytoma is highly suspect but not confirmed after multiple determinations of urinary catecholamines, metanephrines, and VMA, and plasma catecholamines, a test using the central adrenergic blocking agent clonidine has been suggested (protocol p. 208). Plasma catecholamines are drawn (using appropriate precautions to minimize physiologic increases and pharmacologic interferences) before giving clonidine 0.3 mg orally. The patient is kept resting and recumbent and a repeat sample drawn 3 hours later. Clonidine should suppress secretion of norepinephrine from the autonomic nervous system but have no effect on norepinephrine from a pheochromocytoma. There are hazards to this test (particularly postural hypotension), and false-negative and false-positive results may be seen.

A number of drugs interfere with measurement of urine or plasma tests for pheochromocytoma (Table 7–2). In addition to physiologic and pharmcologic circumstances that truly elevate

Table 7–2. Common Interferences with Catecholamine Measurements

False Positives
  Physiologic/Drug-induced
    stress, hypovolemia, etc.
    vasodilators
    theophylline
    beta blocking agents
    peripheral alpha blocking agents
    clonidine withdrawal
  Methodologic
    Urine catecholamines: L-dopa, alpha methyldopa, metyrosine, labetalol, many sympathomimetic amines (theophylline, isoproterenol, etc.)
    Urine metanephrine: MAO inhibitors, benzodiazepines, phenothiazines
    Urine VMA: chloral hydrate, lithium, nalidixic acid, nicotinic acid, quinidine, quinine, tetracycline, salicylates, sulfa drugs
    Plasma catecholamines: phenoxybenzamine, phentolamine, phenothiazines, MAO inhibitors

False Negatives
  Methodologic
    Urine metanephrine: meglumine, renograffin, other IVP dyes (Hypaque is OK); propranolol
    Urine VMA: clofibrate, disulfiram, MAO inhibitors, mandelamine, phenothiazines, salicyclates

levels of catecholamines and metabolites, drugs that produce false positive tests through methodologic interference are L-dopa, alpha methyldopa, metyrosine, and labetalol (urine catecholamines); phenothiazines and isoproterenol (urine metanephrines); nalidixic acid (urine VMA); phenoxybenzamine, phentolamine, phenothiazines, and MAO inhibitors (plasma catecholamines). False-negative results may occur from x-ray contrast dyes and propranolol (urine metanephrines); clofibrate and phenothiazines (urine VMA).

Once a pheochromocytoma has been diagnosed on clinical and laboratory grounds (and only then), studies should be done to determine the location of the tumor. CT scanning of the abdomen and chest will usually provide the answer. Nuclear scanning can be done but there is limited availability of the isotope (^{131}I-meta-iodo-benzylguanidine or MIBG); this technique appears to be as useful as CT. Selective venous catheterization for measurement of epinephrine and norepinephrine may be done, but appropriate reference ranges for interpretation of results are not available and stress-induced increases of catecholamines during the procedure may cause false-positive results.

Treatment of Pheochromocytoma

Definitive treatment of pheochromocytoma is with surgery, but anesthesia and surgery are dangerous unless meticulous attention is paid to patient preparation. *Blockade of catecholamine synthesis* is the method of choice, using alpha-methyl-paratyrosine (*metyrosine,* Demser) given orally, beginning with 500 mg four times daily and increased to as much as 8 gm/day if needed. Adequate inhibition of synthesis can be achieved in 1 to 2 weeks in most patients. Preoperative treatment with metyrosine has the advantage over receptor blocking drugs of preserving tissue responsiveness to adrenergic agonists, which might be required in the event of intra-or postoperative hypotension. Prior to the availability of metyrosine, preoperative treatment employed receptor blocking agents, drugs that may still be useful in selected circumstances.

Alpha-adrenergic receptor blockade with *phenoxybenzamine* can be achieved with a starting dose of 10 mg orally every 12 hours and increased as needed every 3 to 4 days to achieve relief of signs and symptoms. If intraoperative hypertension occurs or if the patient is having a hypertensive crisis, intravenous *phentolamine* (1 to 5 mg) or nitroprusside may be used. *Beta-adrenergic receptor blockade* with propranolol or related compounds may be necessary if tachycardia or cardiac arrhythmia is present, but should only be used after alpha blockade is complete, since hypertension will result from excess alpha activity unopposed by beta activity. Liberal volume expansion before surgery (including blood transfusion, if necessary) may be needed to compensate for decreased blood volume and minimize intra-and postoperative hypotension.

For malignant or unresectable pheochromocytomas, *radiation* or *chemotherapy* may be considered for palliation. For control of adrenergic symptoms, metyrosine may be used, alone or in combination with adrenergic blocking agents such as prazocin (Minipress), phenoxybenzamine (Dibenzylene), or labetalol (Normodyne, Trandate), with combined alpha and beta blocking effects) given for control of symptoms.

Follow-up of pheochromocytoma should be periodic measurements of urine metanephrines or plasma catecholamines, or both (depending on the clinical setting). Results of following patients using MIBG scans suggest that this is a sensitive indicator of recurrence or metastasis, and that pheochromocytoma is more often a malignancy (40 to 50% of cases) than previously thought.

Beierwaltes WH, Sisson JC, Shapiro B, et al.: Pheochromocytoma is often a malignancy. Clin Res 1985; *33*:874a.

Bravo EL, Gifford RW Jr: Pheochromocytoma: Diagnosis, localization and management. N Engl J Med 1984; *311*:1289–1303.

Bravo EL, Tarazi RC, Fouad FM, et al.: Clonidine-suppression test: A useful aid in the diagnosis of pheochromocytoma. N Engl J Med 1981; *305*:623–626.

Eckfeldt JH, Engleman K: Diagnosis of pheochromocytoma. Clin Lab Med. 1984; *4*:703–716.

Engleman K: Phaeochromocytoma. Clin Endocrinol Metab. 1977; *6*:769–797.

Gitlow SE, Mendelowitz M, Bertrani LM: The biochemical techniques for detecting and establishing the presence of a pheochromocytoma. Am J Cardiol. 1970; *26*:270–279.

Metyrosine for pheochromocytoma. Med Lett Drugs Therap. 1980; *22*:28.

Modlinger RS, Ertel NH, Hauptman JB: Adrenergic blockade in pheochromocytoma. Arch Intern Med 1983; *143*:2245–2246.

Shapiro B, Sisson JC, Lloyd R, et al.: Malignant phaeochromocytoma: Clinical, biochemical and scintigraphic characterization. Clin Endocrinol 1984; *20*:189–203.

Swensen SJ, Brown ML, Sheps SG, et al.: Use of 131-I MIBG scintigraphy in the evaluation of suspected pheochromocytoma. Mayo Clin Proc 1985; *60*:299–304.

Taylor HC, Mayes D, Anton AH: Clonidine suppression test for pheochromocytoma: Examples of misleading results. J Clin Endocrinol Metab 1986; *63*:238–242.

RENIN-ANGIOTENSIN-ALDOSTERONE

Background, Pathophysiology

Secretion of aldosterone is controlled primarily by the renin-angiotensin system; the general scheme is shown in Figure 7–4. *Renin* is a proteolytic enzyme synthesized and stored in juxtaglomerular cells of the kidney, which are located along the afferent arterioles of the glomeruli. The important stimuli for renin release are a decrease in perfusion pressure to the juxtaglomerular apparatus and negative sodium balance. Once released into the circulation, renin hydrolyzes its substrate, angiotensinogen (an alpha globulin that is synthesized in the liver), to produce *angiotensin I.* Angiotensin I is then rapidly converted to *angiotensin II* by angiotensin-converting enzyme (ACE), an enzyme that is abundant in the lung. Angiotensin II stimulates the cells of the zona glomerulosa of the adrenal gland to produce *aldosterone.* (Angiotensin II is also a potent vasoconstrictor.) Aldosterone acts on the renal tubules to promote reabsorption of sodium and excretion of potassium.

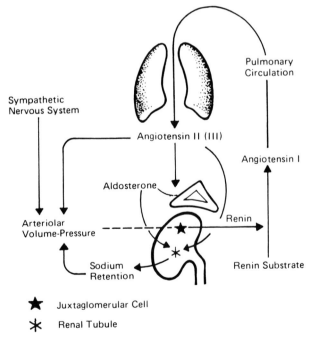

Fig. 7–4. Renin-angiotensin-aldosterone system.

States of Low Renin or Low Aldosterone. Deficient production of aldosterone causes hyponatremia and hyperkalemia, often with hyperchloremic acidosis. Mild or moderate volume depletion may also occur. *Hyporeninemic hypoaldosteronism* is most commonly seen in patients who have diabetes mellitus and mild or moderate renal insufficiency. Demonstrating low plasma renin and aldosterone levels under cirumstances that should cause an increase (furosemide stimulation, upright posture) would be diagnostic.

Clinical Presentation

The interaction of renin, angiotensin, and aldosterone is important in the regulation of extracellular fluid volume, blood pressure, and the balance of sodium and potassium. A change in one of these variables leads to changes in the others. A decrease in effective plasma volume or mean arterial pressure leads to the release of renin from juxtaglomerular cells of the kidneys. More angiotensin is formed, which increases production of aldosterone by the adrenal glands. This results in retention of water and sodium, an increase in extracellular volume, and a decrease in serum potassium. This state of *secondary hyperaldosteronism* is commonly present in congestive heart failure, nephrotic syndrome, cirrhosis of the liver, other hypoproteinemic states, or any condition of chronic depletion of plasma volume. Secondary hyperaldosteronism can be inferred when one of these clinical conditions is observed in patients with volume depletion, edema, and hypokalemic alkalosis. Measurements of renin and aldosterone are seldom needed in these cases.

Primary hyperaldosteronism is characterized by hypertension and hypokalemia, the latter being the result of renal potassium wasting. Since <1% of hypertensive patients have primary aldosteronism, indications that should lead to further evaluation include hypokalemia unprovoked by diuretics, or lack of response to conventional antihypertensive drug treatment. Overproduction of aldosterone may be due to autonomous overproduction of aldosterone by an adenoma of one adrenal gland (aldosterone-producing adenoma or APA, Conn's syndrome), to adrenal carcinoma, or to idiopathic hyperplasia of aldosterone-producing cells in both adrenal glands (idiopathic adrenal hyperplasia, IAH).

Patients with benign essential hypertension may be characterized by plasma renin activity into high (30%), normal (55%), and low (15%) activity. There is disagreement regarding the predictive value of this finding. "Low renin" patients are thought by some to be relatively protected from the increased incidence of cardiovascular complications. Renin measurement may be of some help in the selection of antihypertensive drugs, since most of these agents have predictable effects on renin levels; renin levels do not appear useful for predicting blood pressure response to diuretic treatment, however.

Diagnosis of Hyperaldosteronism

Hypokalemia is the usual clue that primary hyperaldosteronism may be present. If hypokalemia can be shown to be due to nonrenal potassium loss, the diagnosis of primary hyperaldosteronism does not need to be considered further. Figure 7–5 shows a suggested scheme for evaluation of possible hyperaldosteronism in a patient with hypokalemia. Begin by measuring urine potassium when serum is low; urine potassium <30

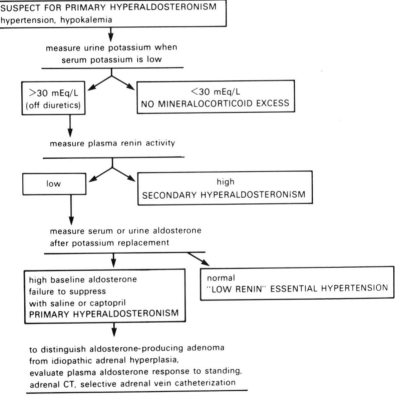

Fig. 7–5. Evaluation for primary aldosteronism.

mEq/L indicates appropriate renal conservation of potassium and rules out mineralocorticoid excess. If renal potassium wasting is present and is due to primary hyperaldosteronism, low renin levels are expected. However, many factors influence basal secretion of renin and aldosterone, and these factors must be recognized and corrected prior to testing. For example, diuretics and upright posture raise plasma renin. Factors that affect plasma renin activity are shown in Table 7–3. Once these factors are eliminated, measurement of plasma renin activity (PRA) is a good initial screening test for primary hyperaldosteronism. Since plasma renin levels vary with sodium balance, it is helpful to compare an individual's ambulatory PRA with his or her level of sodium excretion or to attempt to stimulate renin with a potent diuretic such as furosemide (Fig. 7–6) (protocol p. 211). A low PRA is highly suggestive of primary aldosteronism. A high value, on the other hand, could be due to renovascular disease or pheochromocytoma (secondary hyperaldosteronism).

Once a low PRA has been found in a patient who has hypokalemia due to renal potassium wasting, aldosterone should be measured. The demonstration of an elevated level of aldosterone in blood or urine in a patient with low plasma renin is presumptive evidence for primary hyperaldosteronism. Since hypokalemia has a suppressive effect on aldosterone secretion, the potassium deficit should be replaced before aldosterone measurements are done. To establish autonomous aldosterone overproduction, one may also attempt to suppress aldosterone production with rapid volume expansion (i.e., saline infusion, protocol p. 218) or with a mineralocorticoid such as fludrocortisone (protocol p. 210). Failure of aldosterone to be sup-

Table 7–3. **Factors that Alter Plasma Renin Activity**

Elevation	Reduction
Caffeine	Alpha adrenergic blockers
Captopril	Beta adrenergic blockers
Chlorpromazine	Digoxin
Diazoxide	Indomethacin
Diuretics	Somatostatin
Enalapril	Testosterone
Estrogens	
Guanethidine	
Hydralazine	
Minoxidil	
Nitroprusside	

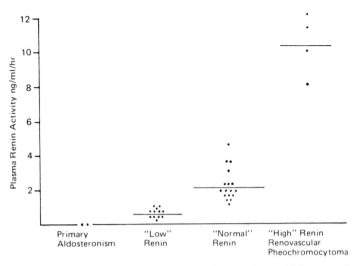

Fig. 7–6. Plasma renin activity after furosemide in patients with hypertension of different etiologies. (Reproduced with permission from Wallach L, Nyari I, Dawson KG: Ann Intern Med 1975; *82*:27–32.)

pressed under these conditions would confirm a diagnosis of primary aldosteronism.

Differential diagnosis of primary hyperaldosteronism is important. Most patients with an aldosterone producing adenoma (APA) respond well to surgical removal of the tumor, whereas patients with idiopathic adrenal hyperplasia (IAH) do not. CT scan localization can help, but some aldosterone-producing tumors are too small to be detected in this way. Iodocholesterol scanning or selective venous sampling for aldosterone may be done. Biochemical clues may help with the differential diagnosis. Aldosterone secretion and plasma renin suppression are usually greater with APA. After sodium restriction and upright posture, patients with APA usually show no change or a fall in plasma aldosterone, whereas patients with IAH typically show a rise in plasma aldosterone.

Plasma renin in *renovascular hypertension* may be useful for case finding (elevated after furosemide stimulation or in relation to urinary sodium excretion) or determining whether surgical treatment would be helpful. Other studies are also useful in this regard. Test selection and treatment of renovascular hypertension are reviewed in a recent article (Working Group on Renovascular Hypertension: Detection, Evaluation, and Treatment of Renovascular Hypertension: Final Report. Arch Intern Med 1987; *147*:820–829.)

Treatment of Hyperaldosteronism

Patients with *idiopathic adrenal hyperplasia* causing primary hyperaldosteronism do not respond well to surgical treatment; the use of *spironolactone,* a mineralocorticoid inhibitor, is usually effective in correcting the hypokalemia but may not be enough to control the hypertension alone. *Treatment of choice for primary hyperaldosteronism due to an adrenal adenoma* is surgical removal, but medical treatment with spironolactone may be tried when the risk of surgery is high.

Kotchen TA, Guthrie GP Jr: Renin-angiotensin-aldosterone and hypertension. Endocrine Reviews 1980; *1*:78–99.

Vaisrub S: Screening for aldosteronism. JAMA 1980; *243*:151–152.

Working Group on Renovascular Hypertension: Detection, evaluation, and treatment of renovascular hypertension: Final report. Arch Intern Med 1987; *147*:820–829.

8

Parathyroid Glands, Kidney Stones, and Osteoporosis

HYPERPARATHYROIDISM

Background, Pathophysiology

There are usually four small parathyroid glands, so named because they lie behind the thyroid gland in the neck. The typical locations are two on each side (left and right)—two at the inferior thyroid poles and two at the superior thyroid poles. Considerable variations from this occur, however. There may be five glands or only three; they may be located almost anywhere within the neck or upper chest. Common aberrant locations are in the tracheoesophageal groove, in the anterior mediastinum attached to the thymus gland, or within the substance of the thyroid itself.

Parathyroid hormone's main role is to maintain normal serum calcium levels. As with most endocrine systems, other factors interact with parathyroid hormone (PTH), particularly vitamin D, magnesium, and calcitonin.

Parathyroid Hormone. Change in the serum calcium concentration seems to be the most important influence on PTH, with increasing release of PTH as serum calcium falls. PTH acts to increase serum calcium in several ways: mobilizing calcium from bone (presumably by increasing osteoclast activity), increasing calcium absorption from the intestinal tract, and increasing calcium reabsorption by the kidney. Phosphorus reabsorption by the renal tubules is reduced by PTH. Vitamin D and magnesium are essential to the normal release and action of PTH, and calcitonin blocks the effect of PTH on bone. All these factors interact to maintain serum calcium in a narrow normal range (Fig. 8–1).

PTH is a polypeptide consisting of 84 amino acids. It is cleaved either on secretion or afterwards, or both, resulting in at least two fragments in addition to the intact molecule being

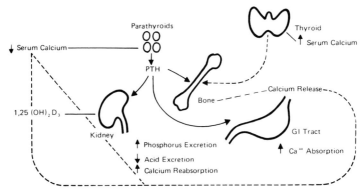

Fig. 8–1. PTH effects and interactions.

present in the circulation. The N-terminal (amino terminal) fragments (amino acids 1-34) have full biologic activity. The C-terminal (carboxy-terminal) fragments (amino acids 35-84) have no biologic activity. PTH exerts its effects at the cellular level through the adenyl cyclase system, and PTH activity is the primary determinant of cyclic AMP found in urine.

A decline in renal function causes a secondary increase in PTH due to the rise in phosphorus and the reciprocal fall in serum calcium. In addition to the expected "secondary hyperparathyroidism," C-terminal PTH fragments accumulate because they are more dependent on renal excretion than N-terminal or intact PTH.

Vitamin D. Just as there are several circulating forms of PTH, there are several circulating forms of vitamin D (Fig. 8–2). The major form is cholecalciferol (vitamin D_3), which is hydroxylated at the 25 position by the liver to produce the more active 25-hydroxyvitamin D_3, and hydroxylated again at the 1 position by the kidney to produce the even more active 1,25-dihydroxyvitamin D_3 (also known as calcitriol). The levels of these substances are determined by liver and kidney function, as well as PTH (which enhances the biosynthesis of 1,25-dihydroxy D) and phosphorus (which inhibits 1 hydroxylation). All are bound to carrier proteins, and the amount of carrier protein will affect the measured value for the total substance. To complicate the issue further, 24,25-dihydroxyvitamin D_3 is present in the blood, but its origin and importance are not clear.

Assays are available for measurement of 25-hydroxy D (normal range 10 to 80 ng/dL) and 1,25-dihydroxy D (normal range 2.1 to 4.5 ng/dL, with higher values in children and late pregnancy). The value of these assays is limited at present by our

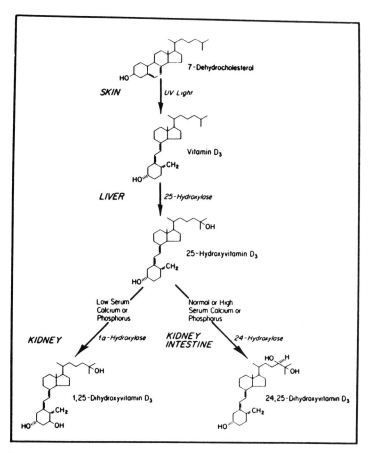

Fig. 8–2. Vitamin D metabolism. (Used with permission from Kumar R, Riggs BL: Vitamin D in the therapy of disorders of calcium and phosphorous metabolism. Mayo Clin Proc 1981; *56*:327–333.)

understanding of the effects that various disease states have on vitamin D metabolism and action (see Aduran M, Kumar R: The physiology and pathophysiology of vitamin D, Mayo Clin Proc 1985; *60*:851–866). 25-hydroxy D levels may be low when levels of the more active 1,25-dihydroxy D are normal and the patient relatively deficient in vitamin D activity. 1,25-dihydroxyvitamin D levels would be expected to be high in primary hyperparathyroidism, as they would in vitamin D toxicity. A normal value would not positively exclude the vitamin D deficient states, osteomalacia or rickets.

139

Clinical Presentation

Primary hyperparathyroidism is the autonomous overproduction of parathyroid hormone. In 85% of cases this is due to a single parathyroid adenoma, but 10 to 15% of cases have hyperplasia of all four glands. Less common causes are multiple (two or three) adenomas or parathyroid carcinoma. The incidence of primary hyperparathyroidism is as high as 1 per 1000, and the ratio of females to males affected is 2 or 3 to 1. The condition is rare in persons under 20 years of age, being seen most frequently in postmenopausal women.

The hallmark of primary hyperparathyroidism is hypercalcemia. There are no specific signs or symptoms. Hypercalcemia may cause polyuria and polydipsia (by interfering with renal concentrating ability), nausea, anorexia, constipation, and alterations in mentation and mood. Hypercalciuria may lead to renal calculi, and prolonged hyperparathyroidism will cause osteopenia due to a reduction in bone mineral content. The clinical presentation in an individual patient depends on the duration and severity of the disease, and ranges from the asymptomatic patient to one with severe multisystem disease.

Causes of Hypercalcemia. There are other causes of hypercalcemia besides hyperparathyroidism. A simple mnemonic ("CHIMPS") lists the common causes of hypercalcemia in relative decreasing order of incidence:

Cancer (including multiple myeloma)
Hyperparathyroidism
Intoxication with vitamin D
Milk-alkali syndrome
Paget's disease of bone (with immobilization)
Sarcoidosis

Other conditions causing hypercalcemia include a variety of drugs (thiazide diuretics, calcium, lithium), hyperthyroidism, adrenal insufficiency, and familial hypocalciuric hypercalcemia.

The most common condition that must be differentiated from primary hyperparathyroidism is hypercalcemia caused by a humoral factor produced by a malignancy, so called *"humoral hypercalcemia of malignancy"* (HHM). Until recently, it was thought by many that these tumors produced PTH, but this does not appear to be the case. Patients with HHM have many but not all of the biochemical features of PTH excess. Similarities include hypercalcemia, hyperchloremic alkalosis, and elevated nephrogenous cyclic AMP, but patients with HHM have low levels of dihydroxyvitamin D, reduced absorption of calcium from the intestine and renal tubules, and impaired bone resorption. There may be several different substances involved in this syndrome, but none are sufficiently similar in structure to PTH to be measured in PTH immunoassays. Recent work indicates that at least one of the substances that mediates HHM shares some structural homology with PTH.

Diagnosis of Hyperparathyroidism

The first step in the diagnosis of hyperparathyroidism is to *demonstrate hypercalcemia.* Finding mild hypercalcemia on a single specimen is suspicious and should be followed up with repeat testing, but is not sufficient for diagnosis. Some patients with hyperparathyroidism will have occasional normal calcium values. Diurnal variation of serum calcium, although slight, makes a morning sample desirable. Elevations due to venous stasis must be excluded, with the sample drawn without venous occlusion if at all possible. Correction must be made for serum protein abnormalities, since calcium is partly bound to serum proteins. Adjusting serum calcium values up or down 0.5 mg for each change in albumin of 1 g, or 0.8 mg for each change in total protein of 1 g is reasonably accurate. Samples should be obtained on several occasions under conditions as ideal as possible. It may be desirable to space the samples over several weeks or months to establish the diagnosis in borderline cases.

Ionized calcium is the metabolically active form of the element and a better indicator of physiologic and pathologic levels of calcium. However, the technique for measurement requires specialized equipment and special care in specimen collection and processing. Reports in the literature suggest the desirability of ionized rather than total calcium measurement when evaluating patients with hyper-or hypocalcemia.

Once the presence of hypercalcemia is established, the process of differential diagnosis begins. The degree of calcium elevation gives some guidance to the diagnostic possibilities:

1. *Marked hypercalcemia* (over 13 mg/dL)—should be treated medically and a nonparathyroid cause should be suspected
2. *Definite hypercalcemia* (11 to 13 mg/dL)—a nonparathyroid cause should be sought; if none is found, operation is indicated
3. *Borderline cases*—repeat measurements to be certain that hypercalcemia is real

Most of the nonparathyroid causes of hypercalcemia should be apparent with a complete history, physical examination, and some simple laboratory tests (CBC; serum albumin, total protein, and creatinine; urinalysis; and chest x ray). In the hands of an experienced surgeon, over 95% of patients with an elevation of serum calcium on three occasions and no evidence of nonparathyroid cause after careful investigation will be found to have hyperfunctioning parathyroid tissue at initial operation.

When the diagnosis of parathyroid disease is suspected, good clinical judgment is still critical. Tests such as nephrogenous cyclic AMP, tubular reabsorption of phosphorus, ratios of chloride to phosphorus, or formulas that include multiple variables have been proposed, but these seem to add little to careful patient selection by excluding other causes of hypercalcemia.

PTH Measurements. Because different forms of PTH circulate in the blood and different antibodies are used in assays for these forms, there has been considerable confusion regarding which PTH assay is "best." The answer is simple: The best assay is the one that correlates best with the clinical condition being sought. So far, no PTH assay has shown uniform elevations in all patients with hyperparathyroidism; with most "good" assays, 10 to 20% of patients with proven parathyroid disease will have "normal" PTH levels. Laboratories that offer PTH measurements should provide the history of the clinical experience of their assay along with patient results. The short half-life of the N-terminal PTH fragment limits the use of this assay in diagnosing hyperparathyroidism; since the C-terminal fragment has such a long half-life, it more closely reflects the amount of hormone secreted by the parathyroid glands, even though the C-terminal fragment has no biologic activity. Since the half-life of the C-terminal fragment is prolonged in renal failure, N-terminal or intact assays are likely to give better information on parathyroid function in patients with renal insufficiency. PTH assays from most laboratories show patients with hypercalcemia due to malignant disease have PTH values generally lower than those seen with hyperparathyroidism; however, about 10% of the PTH values of HHM patients overlap those of patients with hyperparathyroidism, indicating the limited value of the PTH assay for separating hyperparathyroidism from the hypercalcemia of malignancy (Fig. 8–3). Recent improvements in PTH assays offered commercially (by Mayo Medical Laboratories and Nichols Institute) appear to have overcome many of the problems inherent in the older assays. These

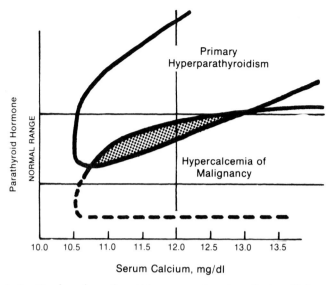

Fig. 8–3. Overlap of parathyroid hormone values in patients with hypercalcemia from malignancy and hyperparathyroidism. (Used with permission from Habener JF, Segre GV: Parathyroid hormone radioimmunoassay Ann Intern Med 1979; *91*:782–783.)

new assays are sufficiently sensitive to detect PTH in most normal individuals. With these assays, PTH values for patients with HHM have been in the low range of normal or below, with little or no overlap with hyperparathyroid patients.

A clearly high PTH level in a patient who has been shown to have hypercalcemia and who has been carefully evaluated for a non-PTH cause is useful confirmation of the diagnosis of primary hyperparathyroidism. If PTH is not diagnostically elevated in a patient who is definitely hypercalcemic, the clinical data should be reviewed and non-parathyroid causes of hypercalcemia sought with extra diligence. PTH measurement should not be done in patients who have normal serum calcium. Patients with metabolic bone disease or recurrent calcium nephrolithiasis should have serum calcium measurements, but, in the absence of hypercalcemia, hyperparathyroidism is unlikely to be present.

A variety of studies are useful for localization of hyperfunctioning or enlarged parathyroid tissue. These include high resolution ultrasound, CT or MR scanning, angiography, selective venous sampling for PTH measurement, and nuclear scanning (thallium-technetium subtraction scans). These studies do not usually help the surgeon doing the initial operation and thus should be reserved for the occasional patient with hyperparathyroidism who requires reoperation for persistence or recurrence.

Treatment of Hyperparathyroidism

Hyperparathyroidism has been diagnosed with increasing frequency and at earlier stages over the past several years, due in large part to the widespread use of automated biochemical profiling. Despite efforts to determine the natural history of mild, "asymptomatic" primary hyperparathyroidism, long-range predictions cannot be made for individual patients. Some seem to do well for many years, while many develop clear indications for intervention (such as renal stones). With thorough evaluation, indicators such as reduced bone density can be found in many otherwise "asymptomatic" patients. In general, most authorities recommend treatment for patients with hyperparathyroidism once the diagnosis is confirmed, although this obviously should take into account the patient's general health and age.

The *treatment of choice* for primary hyperparathyroidism is *surgery.* Since the success rate of surgery depends heavily on the experience and skill of the surgeon, even initial surgery should be done by a surgeon who is very familiar with the anatomic variability of the parathyroid glands. Even if what appears to be an obvious adenoma is identified at first, it should be confirmed by frozen section and the other glands identified, biopsied, and possibly marked with silver clips. Removal of a single adenoma usually results in a cure. Patients with parathyroid hyperplasia are usually treated by removal of all except one-half of a gland; this usually leaves enough parathyroid tissue to maintain adequate PTH secretion for normocalcemia. For patients with hyperparathyroidism due to renal failure (which is always due to hyperplasia) and some with familial hyperparathyroidism, all parathyroid tissue is removed from its normal location and fragments implanted in the muscles of the neck or forearm.

Patients with hypercalcemia persisting after an initial operation for hyperparathyroidism should be referred to a surgeon who specializes in reoperations. Success rates with repeat surgery were in the range of 75 to 80% before localization studies became available and are even higher if patients are studied with CT scans, high-resolution ultrasound, angiography, selective venous catheterization with measurement of PTH, and subtraction scans. Since these studies often give complementary information, it seems advisable to do them all before repeat neck exploration.

Medical treatment may be considered for patients who are not candidates for surgery or refuse operation; however, no medical treatment has been shown to prevent the long-term sequelae of hyperparathyroidism. Estrogen has been shown to normalize serum calcium in many postmenopausal women with hyperparathyroidism. Oral phosphate often lowers symptomatically high calcium to more tolerable levels. PTH antagonists are currently being studied.

Hypercalcemic Crisis

While the best treatment for hypercalcemia is directed at the underlying cause, if the calcium level is dangerously high, acute treatment should be instituted. Most patients with hypercalcemia are dehydrated and show some response to rehydration with normal saline solution. After hydration, the addition of a loop diuretic such as furosemide may lower calcium even further. Other agents used to lower calcium quickly, regardless of etiology, include mithramycin, calcitonin, bisphosphonates, phosphate, glucocorticoids, and indomethacin. The response to most of these agents is unpredictable. Good results are seen with mithramycin, 25 μg/kg IV, which usually normalizes calcium within 12 to 24 hours with the effect lasting for 4 to 7 days; toxic effects may be seen with cumulative doses. Recently, etidronate (a bisphosphonate) has become available for intravenous use. Given in a daily dose of 5 to 7.5 mg/kg/d for several days (along with intravenous saline solution for rehydration), this agent has largely replaced other modalities.

Agus ZS, Wasserstein A, Goldfarb S: Disorders of calcium and magnesium homeostasis. Am J Med 1982; 72:473–488.

Boyd JC, Ladenson JH: Value of laboratory tests in the differential diagnosis of hypercalcemia. Am J Med 1984; 77:863–872.

Burritt MF, Pierides AM, Offord KP et al.: Comparative studies of total and ionized serum calcium values in normal subjects and patients with renal disorders. Mayo Clin Proc 1980; 55:606–613.

Gimlette TMD, Taylor WH: Localization of enlarged parathyroid glands by thallium-201 and technetium-99m subtraction imaging. Clin Nuc Med 1985; 10:235–239.

Habener JF, Segre G: Parathyroid hormone radioimmunoassay. Ann Intern Med 1979; 91:782–785.

Heath H: Tests of parathyroid function: utility and limitations. AACC Endo 1984; 2:1–10.

Hasling C, Charles P, Mosekilde L: Etidronate disodium in the management of malignancy-related hypercalcemia. Am J Med 1987; 82(suppl A):51–54.

Kao PC: Parathyroid hormone assay. Mayo Clin Proc 1982; *57*:596–597.

Lafferty FW: Primary hyperparathyroidism: changing clinical spectrum, prevalence of hypertension, and discriminant analysis of laboratory tests. Arch Intern Med 1981; *141*:1761–1766.

Marx SJ, Stock JL, Altie MF et al.: Familial hypocalciuric hypercalcemia: recognition among patients referred after unsuccessful parathyroid exploration. Ann Intern Med 1980; *92*:351–356.

Mundy GR, Ibbotson KJ, D'Souza SM et al.: Hypercalcemia of cancer: clinical implications and pathogenic mechanisms. N Engl J Med 1984; *310*:1718–1727.

Raisz LG: The diagnosis of hyperparathyroidism (or what to do until the immunoassay comes). N Engl J Med 1971; *285*:1006–1009.

Rude RK, Sharp CF, Freddricks RS et al.: Urinary and nephrogenous adenosine 3',5'-monophosphate in the hypercalcemia of malignancy. J Clin Endocrinol Metab 1981; *52*:765–771.

Scholz DA, Purnell DC: Asymptomatic primary hyperparathyroidism: 10 year prospective study. Mayo Clin Proc 1981; *56*:473–478.

Singer FR, Fernandez M: Therapy of hypercalcemia of malignancy. Am J Med 1987; *82*(Suppl A):34–41.

Suva LJ, Winslow GA, Wettenhall REH: A parathyroid hormone-related protein implicated in malignant hypercalcemia: Cloning and expression. Science 1987; *237*:893–896.

Winzelberg GG: Parathyroid imaging. Ann Intern Med 1987; *107*:64–70.

HYPOPARATHYROIDISM

Clinical Presentation

Hypoparathyroidism most commonly results from neck surgery, but may be idiopathic, due to autoimmune destruction, or due to deficient PTH receptors in target tissues. The main manifestation of hypoparathyroidism is hypocalcemia. Other causes of hypocalcemia include hypomagnesemia (which inhibits release of PTH), vitamin D deficiency, hyperphosphatemia, vitamin D deficiency, sepsis, and pancreatitis. Patients with low serum proteins from malnutrition or other causes often have low total serum calcium but normal ionized values and do not require treatment.

Signs and symptoms of hypocalcemia include evidence of neuromuscular irritability (muscle spasm and cramps, tetany, paresthesias, Chvostek and Trousseau signs), cardiorespiratory embarrassment (bronchial or laryngeal spasm, cardiac arrhythmias, prolonged QT and ST intervals), and CNS problems (irritability, psychosis).

Diagnosis of Hypoparathyroidism

The diagnosis of hypoparathyroidism is usually not a difficult one. If there is any doubt regarding the diagnosis, ionized calcium should be checked (low) and PTH measured (inappropriately low for the hypocalcemia).

Treatment of Hypoparathyroidism

Long-term treatment of the hypoparathyroid patient is best handled with a combination of oral calcium plus a vitamin D preparation, with the doses adjusted based on regular serum calcium measurements to maintain a range of 8.0 to 9.5 mg/dL. In the absence of PTH, calcium alone must be given in high doses. Vitamin D preparations have a narrow therapeutic range. The most commonly used calcium compound is calcium carbonate, which provides more calcium per tablet than lactate or gluconate. Liquid calcium (Neocalglucon) may be used for patients who have difficulty swallowing or absorbing tablets. There are several vitamin D preparations to chose from. Vitamin D_3 (calciferol), usually given in a dose of 50,000 to 200,000 IU/d, has a slow onset of action and, because it is fat soluble, has a long half-life. In patients who develop calciferol toxicity the activity may persist for months after the drug is stopped. 25-Hydroxyvitamin D (calcifidiol), 50 to 200 μg/d, must be converted to dihydroxyvitamin D for full activity, and conversion is impaired in PTH deficiency. 1,25-Dihydroxyvitamin D, 0.25-1.0 μg/d, is a bit more expensive than these other forms, but dose titration appears to be easier. Addition of a thiazide diuretic to reduce renal calcium excretion may permit the use of lower doses of calicum and vitamin D. In some patients with hypoparathyroidism, hyperphosphatemia persists after correcting the serum calcium and a phosphate binder must be added.

Because of the possibility of toxicity, patients with hypoparathyroidism should be followed lifelong with periodic (q 6 to 8 weeks) monitoring of serum calcium.

Hypocalcemic Crisis

Acute treatment of severe, symptomatic hypocalcemia should begin with a bolus of 100 to 200 mg of elemental calcium intravenously over 10 minutes followed by an infusion of calcium at about 1 mg/kg/hr, with the dose adjusted by monitoring the serum calcium level. (A 10-mL ampule of 10% calcium gluconate contains 93 mg elemental calcium; a 10%-ampule of calcium chloride contains 272 mg elemental calcium). When

147

possible, a vitamin D preparation should be added and the route of calcium administration changed from IV to oral. Serum magnesium should be checked and replaced as needed.

Avioli LV: The therapeutic approach to hypoparathyroidism. Am J Med 1974; *57*:34–42.

Harrold CC, Wright J: Management of surgical hypoparathyroidism. Am J Surg 1966; *112*:482–487.

Porter RH, Cox BG, Heaney D, et al.: Treatment of hypoparathyroid patients with chlorthalidone. N Engl J Med 1978; *298*:577–581.

Schneider AB, Sherwood LM: Pathogenesis and management of hypoparathyroidism and other hypocalcemic disorders. Metabolism 1975; *24*:871–898.

Zaloga GP, Chernow B: Hypocalcemia in critical illness. JAMA 1986; *256*:1924–1929.

Zaloga GP,Chernow B: The multifactorial basis for hypocalcemia during sepsis. Studies of the parathyroid hormone-vitamin D axis. Ann Intern Med 1987; *107*:36–41.

RENAL STONES

Patients with renal stones often have abnormalities of urinary constituents that can be identified and treated medically. Many patients have only one kidney stone without recurrences, but patients with two or more stone episodes should be evaluated. Common correctable abnormalities include hypercalciuria (treatable with a thiazide diuretic), hyperuricosuria (treatable with allopurinol), hyperoxaluria (treatable with a low oxalate diet and pyridoxine), and hypocalcitraturia (treatable with oral citrate). Excess urinary uric acid may serve as a nidus for calcium stone formation. Citrate seems to enhance the chemical saturability of urine. Stone analysis may give some clue as to the cause, but 24-hour urinary determination of these four compounds should be done after the patient has recovered from the acute stage of stone passage.

OSTEOPOROSIS

Background, Pathophysiology

Osteoporosis is a major public health problem. Osteoporotic fractures typically involve wedging or compression of vertebral bodies, and breaks of the wrist (Colles fractures) and hip. Fractures of the hip are the most serious consequence of osteoporosis; of the 250,000 hip fracture victims in this country each year, 20% die within a year of complications such as pulmonary emboli or pneumonia, and half the survivors will require long-term nursing care. The estimated total direct and indirect costs of osteoporosis-related fractures in the United States is between 7 and 10 billion dollars a year.

Osteoporosis is a condition of reduced mass of otherwise normal bone, bone that is prone to fracture with minimal stress. A pragmatic definition of osteoporosis requires the presence of a fracture to qualify for the diagnosis; reduced bone mass without fracture is termed "osteopenia." Current diagnostic modalities do not permit an accurate pre-fracture diagnosis of osteoporosis. A number of identifiable disorders and medications are known to accelerate bone loss and lead to "secondary" osteoporosis; "primary" osteoporosis is a diagnosis of exclusion.

Skeletal integrity in adults is maintained through a process called remodeling. Resorption (removal of old bone, mediated by *osteoclasts*) and formation (production of new bone, mediated by *osteoblasts*) are "coupled"; that is, bone formation occurs only after resorption has taken place. After age 30 or 35, an imbalance in these processes (either reduced bone formation, or increased bone resorption, or both) leads to a net loss of bone mineral. Some loss of bone mineral occurs as a result of aging, so the "fracture threshold" (the hypothetical level of bone density below which fractures may occur with minimal trauma) will be reached in everyone who lives long enough. This fracture threshold will be passed early in people whose peak bone mass was low, or if bone loss is accelerated (due to either reduced formation or to increased resorption). Until menopause, rates of bone loss are similar in males and females; however, since women have a 30% lower peak bone mass than men, women reach the point of skeletal instability much earlier than men. This is compounded by the accelerated bone loss occurring in women around the time of menopause (Fig. 8–4). Rapid bone loss affects primarily trabecular bone, which has a much greater surface area than cortical bone. The disparity in rates of loss of trabecular vs cortical bone leads to a predisposition to fractures of bones that are primarily trabecular bone: the vertebral bodies and the wrists. Hip fractures tend to occur later, probably due to the additional loss of cortical bone.

Bone remodeling is influenced by mechanical, electrical, chemical, and hormonal factors. Estrogen deficiency appears to be the major factor in the development of "postmenopausal" osteoporosis. Weight bearing exercise helps preserve bone mass, and activity tends to be less in older individuals. However, excessive exercise has an adverse effect on bone mass;

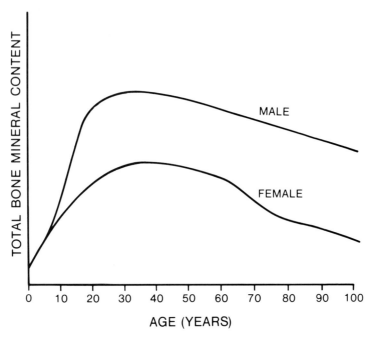

Fig. 8–4. Trends of bone mineral loss in males and females. Reprinted with permission from Watts NB. Osteoporosis. Am Fam Physician (in press). Copyright 1988 American Academy of Family Physicians.

Table 8–1. Risk Factors for Osteoporosis

Age	Race (fair skin)
Sex	Early menopause
Nulliparity	Smoking
Alcohol	Body weight (slender build)
Inactivity	Family history of osteoporosis
Low calcium intake	

women who exercise to the point of developing amenorrhea have been found to have a reduced bone mass for age. Intestinal calcium absorption decreases with age, due in part to diminished production of 1,25-dihydroxyvitamin D. Since dietary calcium intake also decreases with age, many elderly individuals are in a state of negative calcium balance. Increased parathyroid hormone with age appears to be secondary to the changes in vitamin D metabolism and calcium absorption.

Clinical risk factors for osteoporosis are summarized in Table 8–1. For any given age, bone mass is greater in males than females, and greater in blacks than whites. Osteoporosis affects females much more often than males, and only rarely affects blacks.

Clinical Presentation

Osteopenia is often asymptomatic. Not infrequently, reduced bone mineral content is observed on a standard chest x ray in the absence of fractures. Whether this should be called "osteopenia" or "osteoporosis" is debatable. In some women, painless, progressive anterior wedging of thoracic vertebrae leads to loss of height and the "dowager's hump." In others, the first symptom is severe pain due to an acute compression or wedge fracture of a vertebral body (typically T-8 through L-2). Finally, chronic pain due to muscle spasm may persist long after fractures have healed.

Diagnosis and Evaluation of Osteoporosis

Any patient who presents with osteoporosis should be evaluated for the secondary causes that are shown in Table 8–2. Evaluation should begin with a careful history: assessment of location, severity, and character of discomfort; use of analgesics; specific questioning about dietary calcium intake; age at menopause; previous treatment with glucocorticoids, thyroid hormone, or anticonvulsants; and complete physical examination (including documentation of spinal contours and an accurate measurement of height). Laboratory tests should be limited to a screening chemistry panel and complete blood count, unless specific diseases are suspected or suggested by the initial studies. In specific instances, other tests, such as thyroid function, serum or urine protein electrophoresis, measurements of vitamin D metabolites, parathyroid hormone, or urine calcium excretion may be appropriate. Standard lateral radiographs of the spine should be done to document existing fractures, with quantitation of the number and degree of compressions or wedging.

Bone Density Determinations. Standard radiography is in-

Table 8–2.   Secondary Causes of Osteoporosis

Osteomalacia	Hypercalciuria
Alcoholism	Hyperparathyroidism
Metastatic carcinoma	Hyperthyroidism
Multiple myeloma	Cushing's, steroid Rx
Severe liver disease	Hypogonadism
Severe renal disease	Hyperprolactinemia
Malabsorption	Anorexia nervosa

sensitive and cannot be used for early diagnosis of osteoporosis; 30 to 40% of bone mineral must be lost to be detected on routine x rays. Noninvasive techniques are now widely available and in general clinical use, though there is not yet a consensus regarding their appropriate applications. Three caveats should be kept in mind when interpreting the results of bone density measurements: (1) bone density is not the same as bone strength (i.e., factors other than mineral content contribute to fractures), (2) bone density in one site may not correlate with another (e.g., the wrist may be normal while the vertebrae are reduced, or vice versa), and (3) a single measurement cannot define rate (i.e., someone with a "normal" bone density may be losing bone rapidly, while someone with a slightly reduced bone density may be losing bone slowly or not at all).

Experience has shown that measurements of the appendicular skeleton, no matter how precise, do not correlate with bone density of the axial skeleton, so methods such as single photon absorptiometry (SPA) are not useful clinically for the diagnosis or management of osteoporosis. Two methods are applicable to measurement of spinal bone density: *quantitative computed tomography* (QCT) and *dual photon absorptiometry* (DPA). Both methods are accurate (1 to 3%), reproducible (2 to 5%), and moderately expensive (typical charge to the patient at this writing, $150 to $300). Radiation exposure is higher with QCT than DPA (QCT involves 150 to 300 mrem, DPA 1 to 2 mrem, while a standard chest x ray is 70 to 100 mrem). QCT can be used to measure areas of purely trabecular bone in the midportion of the vertebral bodies, while DPA measurements include the cortical bone of the vertebrae as well as spinous and transverse processes.

Despite their individual accuracy and precision, the two methods do not correlate well with each other. With regard to prediction of fracture risk, QCT levels correlate weakly with the prevalence of spinal compression fractures, while DPA levels do not correlate at all. Women with vertebral compression fractures tend to have lower spinal bone mineral content than age-matched controls, though there is a great deal of overlap of bone density measurements by DPA or QCT between women with fractures and those without. Furthermore, subjects with hip fractures do not have a reduced femoral bone density (which can be measured by DPA but not QCT) for their age. The role of bone density measurements for routine diagnosis or follow-up of patients with osteoporosis is not clearly established. While bone density measurements cannot be recommended for general screening of asymptomatic patients at this time, they are useful in establishing a baseline for following treatment in patients with established osteoporosis, and in patients with unusual features of osteoporosis (premenopausal women, males) or in conditions in which reduced bone density may occur (such as hyperparathyroidism, and hyperprolactinemia or other hypogonadal states). If a perimenopausal woman is undecided about taking estrogens, knowledge of her bone mineral content might be helpful in making that decision.

Bone Biopsy. Examination of undecalcified bone from the iliac crest provides a quantitative determination of trabecular bone per total bone volume (an objective measure of osteoporosis) and, with tetracycline labeling, permits the calculation of dynamic parameters of bone remodeling (rates of resorption and formation). Biopsy is the only sure way to differentiate osteomalacia from osteoporosis. Bone biopsy is well tolerated by patients but requires specialized equipment and expert analysis and is expensive. Bone biopsy is recommended for patients with unusual features of osteoporosis, such as young women, blacks, or males, and patients who are not responding to treatment.

Chemical Markers of Bone Metabolism. Some chemical parameters reflect bone remodeling: serum alkaline phosphatase (derived from active osteoblasts, a good indicator of bone remodeling, but bone alkaline phosphatase must be separated from isoenzymes from other organs), urinary excretion of hydroxyproline (an amino acid produced from the breakdown of collagen of bone matrix as bone is resorbed, which correlates well with biopsy evidence of bone resorption), and BGP (also known as bone-Gla protein and osteocalcin, the major noncollagen protein in bone matrix, a good marker of osteoblast function). At present, none of these tests seem suitable for routine clinical application.

Treatment of Osteoporosis

Preventive steps should be started at an early age to maximize peak bone mass and retard bone loss. Adequate intake of calcium should be assured, dietary calcium supplemented with calcium tablets, if necessary, to achieve 1000 mg daily in estrogen replete women and 1500 mg daily in estrogen deficient women. A moderately active lifestyle should be beneficial; no data exist to provide specific guidelines on exercise for osteoporosis, but the equivalent of a brisk 30-minute walk 4 to 7 days a week should be a minimum, supplemented by light

153

weight training where possible. Tobacco and heavy alcohol use should be avoided. These preventive measures would be expected to postpone the onset of symptomatic osteoporosis (Fig. 8–5, line C).

Once osteoporosis has developed, care should be taken to avoid mechanical stresses that might lead to fracture and sedative/tranquilizers that might contribute to falls. Hospitalization is sometimes required for patients with the acute fracture syndrome, since reflex ileus may occur and parenteral analgesics are often required. Chronic muscular pain can be reduced by spinal extension exercises and the judicious use of spinal support. Long-term use of analgesics and muscle relaxants may be necessary in some patients.

Treatment of established osteoporosis should include the same recommendations for prevention of bone loss: adequate calcium intake, a regular (but careful) program of moderate weight-bearing activity, and avoidance of tobacco and heavy alcohol use seem reasonable general recommendations. It

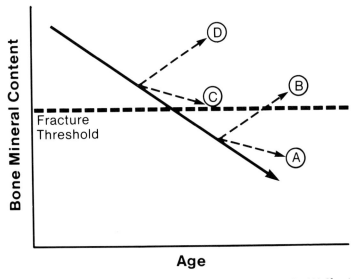

Fig. 8–5. Effect of type and timing of treatment in osteoporosis. (A) Slowing of bone loss when antiresorptive treatment is instituted after overt osteoporosis has developed. (B) How a hypothetical treatment that increases bone mass could eliminate the risk for fracture even after the fracture threshold has been passed. If treatment is begun in high risk patients before the fracture threshold has been reached, antiresorptive agents will postpone fractures (C), while treatment that increases bone mass would prevent the development of osteoporosis (D). Reprinted with permission from Watts NB. Osteoporosis. Am Fam Physician (in press). Copyright 1988 American Academy of Family Physicians.

would seem prudent to take a supplemental multivitamin containing 400 U of vitamin D daily to avoid vitamin D deficiency.

The agents currently approved by the FDA for "treatment" of osteoporosis all work by slowing the resorption of bone, thus reducing the rate of bone loss. These modalities include calcium, estrogen, and calcitonin. In the untreated patient, the risk for fracture, which is already high, increases even more as bone loss continues unabated. These "antiresorptive" agents reduce the risk of future fracture by slowing bone loss, but fail to restore bone mass to a safe level after the fracture threshold has been passed (Fig. 8–5, line A). Instituting antiresorptive therapy in women at risk for osteoporosis while bone mass is still above the fracture threshold (e.g., starting estrogens before accelerated bone loss occurs) (Fig. 8–5, line C) would postpone the time of fracture risk. These agents, though a rational and important part of most treatment programs for most patients with osteoporosis, would not be expected to be of much use after bone loss is far advanced.

Calcium administration would be expected to correct any dietary calcium deficiency, to overcome (at least partially) the impaired calcium absorption that occurs with age, and to reduce parathyroid hormone secretion, secondarily slowing bone resorption. Calcium administration has been shown to reduce the incidence of vertebral fractures in women with osteoporosis. Although recent studies suggest that calcium supplements may not be particularly important in preventing or retarding the accelerated loss of trabecular bone associated with estrogen deficiency, maintenance of adequate calcium intake is hard to argue against. In the absence of contraindications such as hypercalcemia, or patients with calcium-containing kidney stones and hypercalciuria, daily calcium intake should be at least 1000 mg for premenopausal women and women who are taking estrogen and 1500 mg for postmenopausal women not on estrogen. Calcium supplements should be used if dietary calcium is inadequate. Calcium carbonate is well absorbed, and, except for constipation, usually well tolerated.

Estrogens are quite effective in slowing bone loss by reducing bone resorption, probably by inhibiting the response of osteoclasts to parathyroid hormone. When begun at the time of oophorectomy or menopause, estrogen administration has been shown to prevent the expected accelerated bone loss. In women with established osteoporosis, estrogen reduces the risk of vertebral fractures. When used properly, estrogens are not associated with significant risk of breast cancer or endometrial cancer. Clearly, in the absence of such contraindications as hormone-sensitive tumors and thromboembolic disease, estrogens should be given to all women with premature menopause (before age 45), whether surgical or medical. The lowest dose found to be generally effective is 0.625 mg conjugated estrogens daily, though when conjugated estrogen is combined with 1000 mg calcium daily, 0.3 mg daily is equally effective. A woman with an intact uterus should receive estrogen cyclically along with a progestational agent, to reduce the risk of endometrial carcinoma. A typical schedule is conjugated estrogens 0.625 mg days 1 to 25 monthly and medroxyprogesterone 10 mg days 16 to 25 monthly. The addition of a progestational agent may add to the benefits of estrogen on bone. Preliminary work suggests that the combination of daily estrogen and progesterone will lead to endometrial atrophy, which should make hormonal therapy more appealing to women who have looked forward to the absence of menses.

While a fairly good case can be made for the administration of estrogens to all postmenopausal women for prevention of osteoporosis, an even stronger case can be made for estrogens and reduction of the risk of coronary artery disease. Although the effectiveness of estrogens given at the time of menopause is well established, it is not clear what benefits (if any) derive from instituting estrogen 10 years or more after menopause.

Calcitonin is approved by the Food and Drug Administration for treatment of osteoporosis. Pharmacologic doses of calcitonin stop osteoclastic bone resorption, allowing mineralization of existing bone matrix, which leads to an increase in bone density. Studies show an increase in bone mineral content of 10 to 15% with 1 year of treatment with 100 IU calcitonin daily; no further gain (and perhaps some loss) is seen with continued treatment, and bone density returns to baseline levels when treatment is stopped. Most patients who are given calcitonin experience a reduction in pain, apparently due to analgesic properties of the drug.

Calcitonin has not been studied extensively enough to determine whether the slight increase in bone density correlates with a decreased risk of fracture. Calcitonin must be given by subcutaneous injection. Salmon calcitonin is a foreign protein, so allergic reactions or neutralizing antibodies may develop. The use of lower doses (50 IU three times a week), the availability of human calcitonin, and the possibility of intranasal use will overcome some of these drawbacks. Calcitonin is useful for patients with progressive osteoporosis who are not able to take estrogen.

Experimental Therapies

For years, agents have been sought that would restore normal strength to osteoporotic bone (Fig. 8–5, line B) or, if introduced before significant reduction in bone mass has occurred, would prevent osteoporosis and related complications (Fig. 8–5, line D). Research in this field has been difficult because of the lack of suitable animal models and the large number of patients who must be followed to determine fracture rates. Simply demonstrating an increase in bone density after treatment does not assure that bone strength will be improved. Since osteoporosis is a multifactorial disease, there is unlikely to be a single ideal agent. Most of the drugs studied thus far, including calcium, estrogens, and calcitonin, have included significant "non-responder" subgroups. Several approaches are currently being studied that show promise.

Anabolic steroids appear to be moderately effective in increasing bone mass, but are not widely used because of androgenic side effects and toxicity, particularly on the liver.

Vitamin D does not appear to add to the effects of calcium, estrogen, or sodium fluoride. However, active metabolites of vitamin D may be beneficial by increasing bone formation. Problems with interpretation of the current literature on vitamin D metabolites for treatment of osteoporosis include use of different drugs (1-alpha vitamin D, 1,25-dihydroxyvitamin D, 1,24-dihydroxyvitamin D), different doses, and different (and indirect) end points, such as intestinal calcium absorption and urinary calcium excretion, to judge effectiveness. These metabolites appear to reverse the impaired calcium absorption that occurs with aging; whether they can increase bone density and reduce fracture risk remains to be proven. Toxicity is a problem with vitamin D metabolites, with hypercalcemia occurring in many patients. One study suggests that 1,25-dihydroxyvitamin D administration leads to a decrease in vertebral bone mineral content. Until efficacy and safety have been established, treatment of osteoporosis using vitamin D metabolites must be considered experimental.

Sodium fluoride has been studied longest of the drugs in this category. Sodium fluoride appears to work by stimulating function of the osteoblasts, to some degree "uncoupling" bone formation from bone resorption. With high doses of fluoride (>80 mg/day), newly formed bone is histologically abnormal, with

157

wide osteoid seams that suggest osteomalacia. By limiting the dose of fluoride to less than 60 mg daily and giving calcium as well, new bone is formed that is histologically normal. While sodium fluoride treatment increases bone mass and reduces the risk of vertebral fracture in many patients, up to 40% of patients fail to show any response. Although there do not appear to be any serious side effects from the usual therapeutic dose (40 to 60 mg daily), gastrointestinal and rheumatic symptoms have been reported in up to a third of patients treated, severe enough to require stopping the drug in 5 to 10%. Despite these drawbacks, sodium fluoride (plus calcium) is the agent most likely to help patients with progressive osteoporosis. The results of a multicenter, prospective trial of sodium fluoride treatment should be available in the near future and should clarify the role of this agent.

A promising new agent being studied is *1–34 parathyroid hormone (PTH)*, the biologically active part of PTH. In high doses, PTH stimulates bone resorption, but with low doses, bone formation is increased. Combined with 1,25-dihydroxy-vitamin D, 1–34 PTH has been shown to increase bone mass substantially in a small number of patients. This agent must be given by injection and is not generally available. Further studies are needed to determine the safety, efficacy, and optimal doses of this treatment.

Coherence therapy is an intriguing form of treatment for osteoporosis that is currently under investigation at a number of centers, including our own. It relies on manipulation of bone physiology, specifically, the coupling of osteoclast function wtih osteoblast function. Also called A-D-F-R (for *a*ctivate, *d*epress, *f*ree, *r*epeat), coherence therapy is given in a cyclic fashion. One agent is given to activate bone remodeling units and bring them into a resorbing phase (coherence); a second agent is given to depress osteoclastic bone resorption. The osteoblasts are then left free to form new bone before the cycle is repeated. The result is more bone gained per remodeling unit and more remodeling units that are actively forming bone. A number of different drugs could be used in combination for this purpose: possible "activators" include parathyroid hormone, 1,25-dihydroxyvitamin D, thyroid hormones, and phosphate; potential "depressors" are diphosphonates, calcitonin, and estrogens. Studies thus far are encouraging but additional work is necessary to determine the best combination and schedule.

Aloia JF, Cohn SH, Vaswani A, et al.: Risk factors for postmenopausal osteoporosis. Am J Med 1985; *78*:95–101.
Anderson C, Cape RDT, Crilly RG, et al.: Preliminary observations of

a form of coherence therapy for osteoporosis. Calcif Tissue Int 1984; *36*:341–343.

Bikle DD: Fluoride treatment of osteoporosis: A new look at an old drug. Ann Intern Med 1983; *98*:1013–1015.

Cummings SR: Are patients with hip fractures more osteoporotic: Review of the evidence. Am J Med 1985; *78*:487–494.

Ettinger B, Genant HK, Cann CE: Postmenopausal bone loss is prevented by treatment with low-dosage estrogen with calcium. Ann Intern Med 1987; *106*:40–45.

Fatourechi V, Heath H III: Salmon calcitonin in the treatment of postmenopausal osteoporosis. Ann Intern Med 1987; *107*:923–924.

Genant HK, Cann CE, Ettinger B, et al.: Quantitative computed tomography of vertebral spongiosa: a sensitive method for detecting early bone loss after oophorectomy. Ann Intern Med 1982; *97*:699–705.

Hall FM, Davis MA, Baran DT: Bone mineral screening for osteoporosis. N Engl J Med 1987; *316*:212–214.

Health and Public Policy Committee, American College of Physicians: Radiologic methods to evaluate bone mineral content. Ann Intern Med 1984; *100*:908–911.

Ray WA, Griffin MR, Shaffner W, et al.: Psychotropic drug use and the risk of hip fracture. N Engl J Med 1987; *316*:363–369.

Heaney RP, Recker RR, Saville PD: Menopausal changes in calcium balance performance. J Lab Clin Med 1978; *92*:953–963.

Hillner BE, Hollenberg JP, Pauker SG: Postmenopausal estrogens in prevention of osteoporosis: benefit virtually without risk if cardiovascular effects are considered. Am J Med 1986; *80*:1115–1127.

Magos AL, Brincat M, Studd JWW, et al.: Amenorrhea and endometrial atrophy with continuous oral estrogen and progestogen therapy in postmenopausal women. Obstet Gynecol 1985; *65*:496–499.

Riggs BL, Melton LJ III: Evidence for two distinct subtypes of involutional osteoporosis. Am J Med 1983; *75*:899–901.

Riggs BL, Wahner HW: Bone densitometry and clinical decision making in osteoporosis. Ann Intern Med 1988; *108*:293–295.

Riggs BL, Wahner HW, Melton LJ III, et al.: In women dietary calcium intake and rates of bone loss are not related. J Bone Metab Res 1986; *1*(suppl 1):167A.

Riis B, Thomsen K, Christiansen C: Does calcium supplementation prevent postmenopausal bone loss. A double-blind, controlled clinical study. N Engl J Med 1987; *316*:173–177.

Ross PD, Wasnich RD, Vogel JM: Detection of prefracture spinal osteoporosis using bone mineral absorptiometry. J Bone Mineral Res 1988; *3*:1–11.

Slovik DM, Rosenthal DI, Doppelt SH, et al.: Restoration of spinal bone in osteoporotic men by treatment with human parathyroid hormone (1–34) and 1,25-dihydroxyvitamin D. J Bone Mineral Res 1986; *1*:377–381.

9

Diabetes Mellitus and Hypoglycemia

DIABETES MELLITUS

Background, Pathophysiology

Normally, the concentration of glucose in blood is maintained in the narrow range necessary for good health by the interaction of hormones that have opposing effects. *Insulin,* a protein hormone produced in the beta cells of the pancreatic islets, acts to lower blood glucose in two ways: (1) decreasing the production of glucose by the liver, and (2) increasing the entry of glucose into peripheral tissues such as liver, muscle, and adipose tissue. The action of insulin to lower blood glucose can be countered by three means: (1) dietary intake of carbohydrate, (2) production of glucose from other fuels (gluconeogenesis), and (3) release of glucose from glycogen (glycogenolysis). Hormones that elevate blood glucose include glucagon, which is produced by the alpha cells of the pancreas; epinephrine, produced by the adrenal medulla; cortisol, produced by the adrenal cortex; and growth hormone, produced by the pituitary gland. These hormones are referred to as *counterregulatory hormones* because they counteract the effect of insulin on blood glucose. Table 9–1 lists these hormones and their major sites of action. Somatostatin, another pancreatic hormone, is produced by delta cells in the pancreatic islets and modulates the release of insulin and glucagon.

Table 9–1. Counter-regulatory Hormones

	Liver		Muscle		Adipose Tissue	
	Glycogen[a]	Gluconeogenesis	Glucose Uptake	Amino Acid Release	Glucose Uptake	Lipolysis
Growth Hormone	+	+	−	?	−	+
Glucocorticoids	+	+	−	+	−	+[b]
Epinephrine	−	+	−	−[c]	?	+
Glucagon	−	+	0	?	0	?

[a]Net effect on glycogen content via glycogen synthesis or glycogenolysis.
[b]A permissive role.
[c]A β-adrenergic effect, common to several β-adrenergic agonists.
+ = Stimulation or increase; − = inhibition or decrease; 0 = no effect; ? = uncertain
From Ganda OP, *in* Marble A, Krall LP, Bradley RF, et al. (eds.): Joslin's Diabetes Mellitus. 12th ed, Philadelphia, Lea & Febiger, 1985.

Inside the beta cell of the pancreas, a large molecule known as *proinsulin* is formed (Fig. 9–1). Normally only a small amount of proinsulin is secreted into the blood stream. Before secretion, proinsulin is cleaved at two sites, resulting in a biologically inactive protein called connecting or *C-peptide,* and insulin, which consists of two protein chains connected by disulfide bonds. Insulin and C-peptide are released into the portal circulation in equimolar amounts. However, because of the long half-life of C-peptide, the molar ratio of C-peptide to insulin in peripheral blood is about 5 to 1. Since C-peptide is chemically different from insulin, it can be measured by radioimmunoassay even in the presence of circulating antibodies to insulin.

Hyperglycemia is characteristic of diabetes mellitus. Diabetes mellitus is a heterogeneous disorder. In the earliest stages blood glucose is normal but there is an absolute or relative deficiency of insulin—impairment of insulin secretion or insulin action,

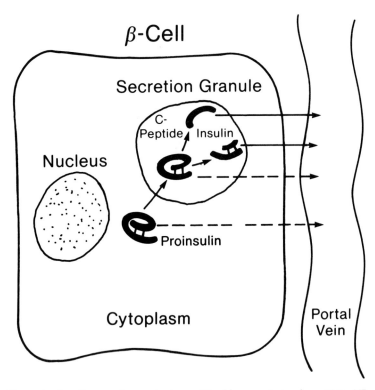

Fig. 9–1.   Insulin secretion and release. (Used by permission from Watts NB, Disorders of Glucose Metabolism. Chicago, ACSP Press, 1987.)

or both. Then, hyperglycemia occurs, initially only after eating due to impaired peripheral utilization of glucose; with progression of the defect, hyperglycemia persists in the fasting state because of unrestrained production of glucose by the liver. Other metabolic abnormalities also result. Over a period of years, patients with diabetes mellitus are prone to develop tissue damage, including accelerated atherosclerosis and relatively specific microvascular changes in the eyes, kidneys, and nerves. Speculation on the exact mechanism(s) of these complications focuses on glycosylation of proteins and accumulation of sorbitol in affected tissues. Regardless of how these complications develop, evidence indicates that diabetic complications correlate with the degree and duration of hyperglycemia. It is hoped that long-term control of hyperglycemia will prevent, or at least minimize, the vascular complications of diabetes.

Table 9–2 shows the classification of hyperglycemia and other categories of glucose intolerance that has been in use since 1979. Diabetes mellitus includes three important types: type I, or insulin-dependent diabetes (IDDM); type II, or noninsulin-dependent diabetes (NIDDM); and gestational diabetes (GDM). Less frequent are "other types" of diabetes, in which hyperglycemia can be attributed to a specific underlying disorder such as chronic pancreatitis or Cushing's syndrome. Impaired glucose tolerance includes subjects who have blood glucose values that are somewhat higher than normal but not high enough to be a reliable indicator of diabetes. The last two categories are useful primarily to researchers—previous abnormality of glucose tolerance refers to subjects who had abnormal glucose tolerance in the past but are normal at the time of study, and potential abnormality of glucose tolerance, in which blood glucose is normal but diabetes is considered likely to develop because of a strong family history or other reasons.

Table 9–2. Classification of Diabetes and Other Categories of Glucose Intolerance

Diabetes Mellitus (DM)
    Type I, insulin-dependent diabetes mellitus (IDDM)
    Type II, noninsulin-dependent diabetes mellitus (NIDDM)
    Other types, attributable to underlying disorders
Impaired Glucose Tolerance (IGT)
Gestational Diabetes (GDM)
Previous Abnormality of Glucose Tolerance (PrevAGT)
Potential Abnormality of Glucose Tolerance (PotAGT)

Type I diabetes mellitus is also called insulin-dependent diabetes or IDDM. Diabetes develops because of autoimmune destruction of the beta cells. Circulating antibodies against beta cells are present at the time of diagnosis in over 90% of subjects with IDDM. These antibodies, and the subsequent development of diabetes, are much more likely to occur in individuals who have the genetic susceptibility associated with specific HLA types (DR3, DR4). IDDM patients have a near total deficiency of insulin and depend on the administration of insulin to stay alive. If insulin is not given, severe hyperglycemia and diabetic ketoacidosis develop. The onset of type I diabetes usually occurs in childhood or adolescence but it may develop at any age. Former terms for type I diabetes include juvenile diabetes, ketosis-prone, or brittle diabetes.

Type II diabetes mellitus is also known as noninsulin-dependent diabetes or NIDDM. This is the most common form of diabetes, comprising 85 to 90% of all patients with diabetes, and affects some 12 million Americans. Most patients with type II diabetes are obese. Type II diabetes is due at least in part to impaired insulin action, but insulin deficiency also plays a part. Some patients have high levels of insulin in blood; in others, insulin is normal, and in others, insulin is low. The presence of even small amounts of insulin protects these patients from the development of ketosis in the basal state. Some patients with type II diabetes need insulin treatment to control hyperglycemia. The onset of type II diabetes usually occurs after age 40, but it may occur at any age. Former terms for type II diabetes include adult-onset or maturity-onset diabetes, ketosis-resistant diabetes, and a subset of young people with type II diabetes called maturity onset diabetes of youth, or M-O-D-Y.

In NIDDM the causes of hyperglycemia are several. The beta cells do not release insulin appropriately in response to hyperglycemia. In many NIDDM patients, although insulin release is delayed, total insulin secretion is greater than normal. Why should an individual with elevated insulin levels become hyperglycemic? The answer lies in impairment of insulin action in its target tissues. When insulin is present in normal or increased amounts but fails to demonstrate normal action, this is referred to as *insulin resistance.* For insulin to exert its effects, it must first be transported through the blood, then bind with receptors on the cell surface. It is known that the number of insulin receptors decreases as the concentration of insulin increases (down regulation). Insulin levels are increased in obesity, and insulin receptors are decreased in many target sites in obese subjects. If such an individual has a limited capacity to produce insulin, the result will be hyperglycemia. These changes in insulin receptors are reversible; with weight loss, insulin levels are reduced and insulin receptor number increases.

Insulin resistance is more than changes in insulin receptors. After insulin binds with its receptor, events are initiated within the cell that result in insulin action. These intracellular changes are not yet well defined, and are referred to generally as "post-receptor" or "post-binding" events. Most obese patients with NIDDM have a significant component of insulin resistance due to postreceptor defects or receptor changes, or both.

Gestational diabetes refers to the onset of glucose intolerance during pregnancy. The cause of GDM is not known, but it is probably a combination of impaired insulin secretion (similar to NIDDM) and resistance to insulin action caused by the counter-insulin action of placental hormones. It is clear that untreated gestational diabetes is associated with increased perinatal complications such as high birth weight infants, respiratory distress syndrome, hypoglycemia, and jaundice. Detection of gestational diabetes is quite important, since control of maternal hyperglycemia has been shown to substantially reduce or eliminate these risks to the infant. Though most women with gestational diabetes will revert to normal glucose tolerance after delivery, 30 to 50% will develop type II diabetes after 10 years. Patients should be retested and reclassified after pregnancy.

Clinical Presentation

Patients with *IDDM* usually come to the physician's office or emergency room with clear-cut hyperglycemia, often with ketoacidosis and symptoms and signs that demand attention. There is some promise from research that high-risk subjects can be identified before the development of ketoacidosis by the presence of circulating islet-cell antibodies or changes in insulin secretion, and perhaps treated with immunosuppressive drugs to prevent islet cell destruction. These techniques are not yet ready for general application.

The onset of *NIDDM* is usually more gradual than IDDM, and the symptoms are more subtle. Often, NIDDM is diagnosed when "routine" laboratory studies reveal an elevated glucose. Symptoms, if present, may include polyuria, polydipsia, dry mouth, blurred vision, fatigue, and weight loss. Urinary tract infection or monilia vaginitis may be present. Occasionally, NIDDM is first recognized in patients presenting with complications of atherosclerosis (coronary ischemia, stroke, lower extremity vascular insufficiency).

GDM is usually a laboratory diagnosis. Factors indicating a high risk for gestational diabetes include glycosuria, obesity, a history of large babies, unexplained neonatal death or stillbirths, habitual abortions, hydraminos, and a family history of diabetes.

Diagnosis of Diabetes Mellitus

The diagnosis of *IDDM* is usually apparent when the patient has the abrupt onset of suggestive symptoms and signs (polyuria, polydipsia, dehydration) and is readily confirmed by a definite elevation of serum glucose (>200 mg/dL). Although other tests are indicated for evaluation of the patient, no further diagnostic measures are needed.

The diagnosis of *NIDDM* may be made by finding a significantly elevated postprandial (>200 mg/dL) or fasting (>140 mg/dL) serum glucose. The oral glucose tolerance test (OGTT) is usually not needed and can present problems. The criteria for OGTT interpretation used before 1979 were not specific enough to be predictive; that is, abnormal tests occurred in patients without diabetes. Criteria were revised in 1979; these criteria are shown in Table 9–3 and should be used if an OGTT is done. NIDDM is confirmed by OGTT if the 2-hour value is above 200 mg/dL *and* one other value is greater than 200 mg/DL.

Conditions to be met for a valid OGTT are shown in Table 9–4. Only healthy, ambulatory subjects should be tested—it is *not* a test for hospital inpatients. At least 3 days of unrestricted diet and activity should precede the test; the diet should contain at least 150 g of carbohydrate a day. Medications known to impair glucose tolerance, such as diuretics, estrogens, or steroids, should be stopped. The oral glucose load for the diagnosis of NIDDM in adults is 75 g (100 g is used for GDM). The test for NIDDM is a 2-hour test, with samples drawn fasting, 1 hour, and 2 hours being sufficient for most purposes (protocol p. 212);

Table 9–3. Criteria for the Diagnosis of Diabetes Mellitus in Nonpregnant Adults

A. Random plasma glucose >200 mg/dl OR
B. Fasting plasma glucose >140 mg/dl OR
C. Abnormal oral glucose tolerance test:
   serum glucose >200 mg/dL at 2 h *and*
   >200 mg/dL at 1 h

Table 9-4.   Conditions To Be Met For a Valid Oral Glucose Tolerance Test

Healthy, ambulatory subjects (not a hospital test)
Stop drugs known to impair glucose tolerance
3 days of unrestricted diet and activity (at least 150 g carbohydrate daily)
Test in AM after 10 to 16 hour fast
75 g oral glucose solution
Venous plasma glucose fasting, 1 and 2 hours, or fasting, 30, 60, and 90, and 120 min
No need for urine glucose measurements

From Watts NB: Disorders of Glucose Metabolism, ASCP Press, Chicago, 1987.

sampling every 30 minutes for 2 hours is recommended for research studies.

When an OGTT is done, some individuals will have glucose values that are higher than normal but not high enough to meet the criteria now accepted for the diagnosis of NIDDM (Table 9–3). These individuals fall in the category of *impaired glucose tolerance (IGT)*. Fasting serum glucose will be normal, otherwise the patient would have NIDDM. A 2-hour glucose result between 140 and 200 *and* one other value over 200 would meet the criteria for impaired glucose tolerance. There is a high probability that an individual in this group will revert to normal or remain in this intermediate range. Patients in this category show a slow rate of progression to overt diabetes, between 1 to 5% each year. As a group, there is an increased risk for cardiovascular disease; IGT is a risk factor similar to cigarette smoking or an increased blood cholesterol. However, those patients who progress from IGT to NIDDM have a low risk of developing microvascular disease.

All pregnant women should be screened for *gestational diabetes* (GDM) in the first trimester. Screening can be done at any time of the day, without regard for previous meals, by measuring serum glucose after an oral glucose load. A 50-g glucose load is given; serum glucose >140 mg/dL 1 hour later is positive (protocol p. 211). Women with a positive screening test should have an oral glucose tolerance test. Since glucose tolerance deteriorates during the last trimester of pregnancy, high-risk women with a normal screening test or GTT in the first trimester should be retested at about 32 weeks' gestation.

The OGTT for GDM is a 3-hour test, with serum glucose measured fasting and hourly for 3 hours after administration of 100 g of an oral glucose solution (protocol p. 212). The results are interpreted using the criteria of O'Sullivan and Mahan published in 1964 (Table 9–5).

Table 9–6 reviews the glucose tolerance tests for NIDDM and GDM. For NIDDM, it is a 2-hour test using a 75-g glucose load. The 2-hour value is the most important one; if it is over 200 mg/dL, diabetes can be diagnosed. If the 2-hour value is between 140 and 200, the patient should be classified as having impaired glucose tolerance. For GDM, the OGTT is a 3-hour test using a 100-g glucose load. At least two values must exceed the levels shown. Remember that for NIDDM or GDM, screening tests should be done before an OGTT is ordered and that standard conditions for testing shown in Table 9–4 must be met.

Treatment of Diabetes Mellitus

Education of patients is the cornerstone of good diabetes management. Proper diabetes education requires a health professional (usually physician or nurse) who has training and experience in diabetes treatment, as well as the time and communication skills to teach and motivate patients. The more complicated the treatment program, the more essential good diabetes education is.

It has been said, "the secret of a long life is to get a chronic

Table 9–5. Criteria for the Diagnosis of Gestational Diabetes Mellitus

Two or more of the following venous plasma glucose values must be met or exceeded:
fasting, 105 mg/dL
one-hour, 190 mg/dL
two-hour, 165 mg/dL
three-hour, 145 mg/dL

From O'Sullivan and Mahon, Diabetes, 1964; *13*:278.

Table 9–6. Comparision of Glucose Tolerance Tests for NIDDM, IGT, and GDM. (Results are reported as plasma glucose in mg/dL)

Time (hours)	NIDDM (2-hour test, 75 g glucose)	IGT	GDM* (3-hour test, 100 g glucose)
0		<140	105
1	>200	>200	190
2	>200	140–200	165
3	—	—	145

*At least 2 values should exceed these levels.
Reproduced by permission from Watts NB: Disorders of Glucose Metabolism, ACSP Press, Chicago, 1987.

disease and then take good care of yourself." Everyone should follow *good health habits,* especially patients with diabetes. These include regular physical activity for optimal physical fitness; a sensible diet with moderate or low intake of sodium, high fiber, low cholesterol, high polyunsaturated fat; and maintenance of desirable body weight.

Proper eating (or "diet") is advisable for patients with diabetes. There are three general principles: (1) limit sweets, which raise blood glucose more rapidly than other foodstuffs, (2) eat regular meals, at least three times a day (this is particularly true for patients receiving insulin or an oral hypoglycemic agent); and (3) achieve and maintain a desirable body weight. The latter objective is especially important in NIDDM since most NIDDM patients are obese and obesity contributes to insulin resistance. There are no secrets for successful weight loss, and no single program that is highly effective. The Weight Watchers program emphasizes sensible eating habits and works well for patients who are comfortable in a group setting. Individualized programs are more expensive and should be recommended only on a case-by-case basis. "Fad" diets rarely show long-term effectiveness, probably because they neglect strategies to change the poor eating habits that led to the weight gain in the first place. Instruction by a dietitian in an "ADA" diet (meal planning using a list of exchanges to assure good nutritional balance and estimate calories) should be considered for all patients with diabetes.

Treatment Goals in Diabetes Mellitus

Most authorities agree that normal or near-normal levels of blood glucose are desirable, and with current techniques of monitoring and intensive insulin treatment—by multiple injections or an infusion pump—that most people with diabetes can achieve and maintain tight control. There is evidence from extensive animal studies and some work in man that normalization of blood glucose *before* diabetic complications develop will reduce or eliminate these complications. Tight control is an ideal goal, but individual circumstances may be present that indicate that a higher blood glucose level than normal may be acceptable or desirable. These include a tendency toward severe hypoglycemia, older age (less time for hyperglycemia to do damage), or inadequate support or abilities (intellectual, motivational, financial) to work with a program of intensive treatment. Once the diagnosis of diabetes is made, a plan for treatment must be instituted, and the effectiveness of treatment must be assessed.

Monitoring

A variety of ways exist to assess control of diabetes. Clinical signs and symptoms of high or low blood glucose are insensitive and cannot be used to "fine tune" a management program. For years, patients were taught to measure urine glucose and to use their results to adjust treatment. Urine glucose often gives inaccurate information about serum glucose, being negative when serum glucose is high, or elevated when serum glucose is normal. At best, urine glucose measurements can be used in some patients for making gross adjustments in treatment, but urine glucose tests are not sufficiently accurate to be used to achieve tight control. While urine testing for glucose may be outmoded for most patients, *urine ketone* determination still has a role in the monitoring of patients with type I diabetes to detect ketoacidosis.

Several methods for glucose determination on capillary blood samples are now available that are simple and inexpensive enough for patients to do frequent blood glucose determinations on their own. This is the most significant advance in diabetes management since the discovery of insulin. Patients can obtain a capillary blood sample with only slight discomfort using a spring-loaded lancet and test for glucose with one of several reagent strips or systems suitable for reading by visual inspection or reflectance meter.

Self blood glucose testing is useful for all patients with diabetes mellitus and is a prerequisite for achieving and maintaining normal blood glucose levels (tight control). It is particularly useful for patients who are prone to severe hypoglycemic reactions; during pregnancy, when achieving tight control is particularly important; and for individuals who are being treated with an insulin infusion pump or intensive insulin therapy. The results of self blood glucose testing can be analyzed by the patient or physician to detect patterns of high or low glucose so the individual's diabetes treatment regimen can be optimized by making adjustments in insulin dose, diet, or activity. When a patient's schedule varies, blood glucose results can be used to determine the need for supplemental insulin or extra calories. When insulin needs are changing rapidly, such as during illness, frequent blood glucose determinations by the patient, family, or hospital staff are a valuable guide for adjusting the insulin dose. In many hospitals, reflectance meters for rapid glucose testing are being used routinely on the wards.

The desired frequency of self blood glucose testing depends on the specific needs of the patient. Someone striving for tight control will probably need to test before each meal and at bedtime every day, sometimes more often. For a patient with stable insulin requirements or when less meticulous glucose control seems appropriate, "spot checking" a few times a week may be adequate, with daily pre-meal and bedtime profiles done if the spot check results indicate undesirable control. Patients treated with "diet alone" may not need to monitor regularly, but knowing how to test their own blood glucose may save them a doctor visit during illness.

Hemoglobin A_{1c} (glycosylated hemoglobin or HbA_{1c}) is a useful test for monitoring diabetes control and complements the results of self blood glucose testing. HbA_{1c} reflects the patient's average blood glucose for approximately 2 months prior to testing. Glycosylated hemoglobin is formed when carbohydrate combines with hemoglobin; when the carbohydrate is glucose and hemoglobin is the normal adult variety (hemoglobin A) the product is known as hemoglobin A_{1c}. (Some methods give falsely low values in patients with variant hemoglobins such as hemoglobins S or C.) Other carbohydrate-hemoglobin combinations occur, but only in small concentrations. The amount of HbA_{1c} formed is proportional to the mean ambient glucose concentration and the life span of the red cell. When red cell survival is normal (120 days), HbA_{1c} reflects the mean glucose concentration of the previous 2 months. This relationship will vary if red blood cell survival is abnormal.

Glycosylated hemoglobin provides an objective test independent of patient preparation. When HbA_{1c} and patient monitoring results are at variance, usually the problem lies with the patients' accuracy or misrecording of their self blood glucose tests. If patients have not been testing blood glucose at home, HbA_{1c} provides data about their previous level of glucose control. While this test is not sufficiently sensitive for general use in the diagnosis of diabetes, it does have diagnostic significance in one situation: "stress hyperglycemia." If a patient is found to be hyperglycemic during stress, such as on admission to the coronary care unit with a myocardial infarction, an elevated HbA_{1c} is strong evidence that the patient has diabetes and has been hyperglycemic for some time. A normal HbA_{1c} in this setting indicates that hyperglycemia is probably a response to the acute stress and is likely to resolve once the stress is over.

Fructosamine is a test similar to HbA_{1c}. Glucose combines with albumin and other serum proteins to produce glycosylated products; the rearrangement of glucose after combination with an amino acid produces a fructose-amine. In principle, this test should reflect the glucose level over a much shorter period than HbA_{1c}, perhaps 2 or 3 weeks as opposed to 2 months. However, published information on applications of this test is limited. The test result is expressed as an absolute value rather than as percent of the substrate affected; this means that changes in the amounts of albumin or other serum proteins that affect the amount of fructosamine are not reflected in the result. With these caveats, fructosamine measurement may be of some use in evaluating diabetic control.

Insulin

All patients with IDDM and many patients with NIDDM and GDM require insulin to control hyperglycemia. Patients with NIDDM and GDM should not be started on insulin unless glucose fails to reach a satisfactory level with nonpharmacologic treatment (so-called "diet alone," but really multiple efforts including good eating habits, weight reduction, improved physical conditioning, elimination of medications that interfere with insulin action, and self blood glucose monitoring).

Types of Insulin. Animal insulins largely have been replaced by synthetic human insulins. Human insulins have some real and theoretical advantages over animal insulins including an essentially unlimited supply and less antigenicity (circulating antibodies to insulin may alter insulin absorption or action). The price of human insulins is now similar to that of animal insulins, so there is little reason to continue the use of insulins of beef or pork origin. The main decision regarding the type of insulin to use relates to pharmacokinetics: time to peak and duration of action. There are four general categories: (1) very long acting (Ultralente), (2) intermediate acting (NPH and Lente), (3) short acting (Regular and Semilente); and (4) premixed (Mixtard or Novolin 70/30, 7:3 proportions of intermediate and short acting insulin). The characteristics of these insulins are shown in Table 9–7.

Some patients with NIDDM require only a single dose of intermediate acting insulin in the morning or at bedtime. However, most patients with IDDM and GDM (and many patients with NIDDM) require more than one injection of insulin a day ("split dose") and more than one type of insulin ("mixed"). Some patients with unpredictable schedules do best with 40 to

Table 9–7. Characteristics of Different Types of Insulins

	Action (Hours)		
	Onset	*Peak*	*Duration*
RAPID			
Regular	0.2–0.5	2–4	5–7
Semilente	0.5–1	2–6	6–8
INTERMEDIATE			
NPH	1–2	6–12	18–24
Lente	1–2	6–12	18–24
LONG			
Ultralente	4–6	18–24	32–36
PZI	4–6	14–20	24–36

50% of their daily insulin as Ultralente and the remainder as boluses of short-acting insulin before meals (three or four injections a day). For better convenience and compliance, the typical "split-mixed" insulin regimen consists of two injections a day (before breakfast and supper) with two types of insulin (intermediate and short-acting) in each. The actual amounts must be determined for each patient. Total daily insulin requirements can be estimated by multiplying the patient's body weight in pounds by 0.3 Units of insulin; this is divided, with $\frac{2}{3}$ of the total dose before breakfast, $\frac{1}{3}$ before supper; $\frac{2}{3}$ as intermediate, $\frac{1}{3}$ as short-acting. For example, 150 pounds body weight $\times$ 0.3 U = 45 units of insulin a day; divide this up as 20 NPH + 10 Reg q AM, 10 NPH + 5 Reg q PM. Adjustments in these components, 10 to 20% each time, are made as patterns are found in the blood glucose record, using the assumption that each component of the insulin schedule is assessed with one of the four blood tests during the day: AM Regular with pre-lunch blood test, AM NPH with the pre-supper test, PM Regular with bedtime test, and PM NPH at breakfast the next day. For rapid control of unexpected hyperglycemia or calculation of extra insulin for stress or illness, supplements of Regular insulin may be given with amount of the supplement determined with a formula such as ((blood glucose $-100/S$) = Units of Regular insulin to take, where S = (1500/total units of insulin each day)). For example, S in a patient taking 50 Units of insulin a day is 30 (1500/50), so for a blood glucose of 250, the calculation goes as follows: (250–100)/30 = 150/30 = 5 Units of Regular insulin to be taken.

Oral Hypoglycemic Agents

Oral hypoglycemic agents are contraindicated in GDM and are ineffective in IDDM and some patients with NIDDM. These agents appear to work by improving insulin secretion or insulin action or both. Patients with NIDDM who do not achieve satisfactory glucose control with nonpharmacologic measures may respond to oral agents; the best response is seen in patients who are compliant with diet but still obese and only moderately hyperglycemic. Although there are several classes of oral hypoglycemic agents, all those currently approved for use in this country are sulfonylureas. The two "second-generation" drugs introduced a few years ago have fewer toxic effects than the first generation drugs, so one only needs to be familiar with two agents. Glipizide (Glucotrol) (maximum total daily dose 40 mg) is shorter acting than glyburide (DiaBeta, Micronase) (maximum total daily dose 20 mg). The dose should be adjusted to the least amount of medication required to achieve a good therapeutic response. There are no compelling reasons to chose one of these agents over the other. Patients who fail to respond to one usually do not respond to the other and generally require insulin to control hyperglycemia.

Diabetic Ketoacidosis (DKA)

This potentially fatal complication of diabetes requires hospital admission and close monitoring of the patient. It is advisable to create a flow sheet for recording treatment and laboratory results. Look for and treat any precipitating cause. Most patients with DKA are quite dehydrated, averaging a fluid deficit of 6 to 8 L because of urinary losses (the result of osmotic diuresis). Fluid resuscitation should begin with isotonic saline solution given as rapidly as possible, with the rate slowed and changed to hypotonic saline after the first 2 to 3 L. Attention must be given to serum electrolytes. DKA patients are usually quite potassium depleted but because acidosis causes potassium to shift out of cells, serum potassium is often normal or high initially. Potassium replacement should be started as soon as adequate renal function is established (good urine output, normal serum creatinine). Most patients with DKA are also phosphate depleted. However, phosphate replacement has no effect on response to treatment and should not be used routinely. Phosphate administration should be given when serum phosphate is <1.0 mg/dL.

The dose of insulin used to treat DKA should be "enough."

Most patients will respond to 10 U regular insulin per hour given as a continuous IV infusion but the dose should be increased if the acidosis is not clearing. Remember that you are treating *ketoacidosis,* not just hyperglycemia; keep up the insulin infusion until CO_2 and pH are near normal, adding dextrose to IV fluids to prevent hypoglycemia, if necessary.

Diabetes and Surgery

NIDDM patients who are well-controlled with nonpharmacologic or oral agent treatment may be managed through surgery by withholding medication and avoiding intravenous dextrose. Insulin-requiring diabetics can be managed through surgery in a number of ways; IDDM patients should always receive some insulin. Insulin may be given SQ on the morning of surgery as a fraction (⅓, ½, ⅔) of the usual daily dose, with supplements of regular insulin SQ based on blood glucose determinations. If IV dextrose is given, it is best to keep the rate constant.

We have developed a simple algorithm using an insulin infusion, adjusting the infusion rate based on reflectance meter

Table 9–8. Orders for the "Steady State" Insulin Infusion

(1)	IV fluids: D5–0.45% saline @ 100 ml/h, add 20 mEq KCl/L[a]
(2)	Insulin drip: 125 U Regular insulin in 250 ml 0.9% saline[a] (1 ml of solution = 0.5 U insulin, 2 ml solution = 1 U insulin)
(3)	Begin insulin drip at 1.5 U/h (3 ml/h)[b]
(4)	Blood glucose with reflectance meter q 2 h
(5)	Based on blood glucose, do the following: 120–180: no change 181–240: increase insulin drip by 0.5 U/h >240: increase drip by 0.5 U/h *and* give 8 U regular insulin IV 80–119: decrease drip by 1.0 U/h <80: decrease drip by 1.0 U/h *and* give 25 ml D50 IV
(6)	If drip rate is reduced to zero, continue reflectance meter glucose checks q 2 h and restart drip at 0.5 U/h when glucose >150
(7)	Notify physician if glucose <80 or >240 on two consecutive checks[c]

[a]If volume needs to be limited, D10—W @ 50 ml/h should be used as the main IV; KCl concentration should be adjusted to patient needs.

[b]Starting rate may be higher if the patient is known to require high doses of insulin, or lower if the patient is thought to be unusually sensitive to insulin.

[c]If the insulin rate is >6 U/h and glucose control is not steady, adjustments and boluses may need to be in larger increments.

Modified from Diabetes Care 1987;10:722–728. © Nelson B. Watts, 1987.

blood glucose determinations at the bedside (Diabetes Care 1987; *10*:722–728). This protocol is simple enough for use on a general medical or surgical ward yet maintains stable blood glucose control in most patients. Dextrose is given at a fixed rate to minimize the risk of hypoglycemia. The orders for this "steady state" insulin infusion are shown in Table 9–8.

Complications: Recognition and Management

Certain complications occur in many patients with long standing diabetes mellitus. It is thought that these complications relate in large part to the degree and duration of hyperglycemia. Atherosclerosis develops at an earlier age and progresses more rapidly in diabetics than in nondiabetics. Included in these *macrovascular* complications are peripheral vascular insufficiency, coronary atherosclerosis with angina and myocardial infarction, and cerebral atherosclerosis with stroke. *Microvascular* complications are relatively specific for diabetes and include nephropathy, neuropathy, and retinopathy. It is beyond the intended scope of this manual to discuss these complications in detail. Surveillance for these complications is an important part of the follow-up of diabetic patients.

GENERAL

American Diabetes Association: Gestational diabetes mellitus. Ann Intern Med 1986; *105*:461.
Cryer PE: Glucose counterregulation in man. Diabetes 1981; *30*:261–264.
Davidson JK (ed.): Clinical Diabetes Mellitus: A Problem Oriented Approach. New York, Thieme, Inc., 1986.
Eisenbarth GS: Type I diabetes mellitus: A chronic autoimmune disease. N Engl J Med 1986; *314*:1360–1368.
Freinkel N, Dooley SL, Metzger BE: Care of the pregnant woman with insulin-dependent diabetes mellitus. N Engl J Med 1985; *313*:96–101.
Gerich JE: Insulin-dependent diabetes mellitus: pathophysiology. Mayo Clin Proc 1986; *61*:787–791.
Kahn CR: Insulin receptors and syndromes of insulin resistance. Diabetes Care 1982; *5*(Suppl 1):98–101.
Krolewski AS, Warram JH, Rand LI, et al.: Epidemiologic approach to the etiology of type I diabetes mellitus and its complications. N Engl J Med 1987; *317*:1390–1398.
Marble A, Krall LP, Bradley RF, et al. (eds.): Joslin's Diabetes Mellitus, 12th ed. Philadelphia, Lea & Febiger, 1985.
National Diabetes Data Group: Classification and diagnosis of diabetes mellitus and other categories of glucose intolerance. Diabetes 1979; *28*:1039–1057.
Service FJ: What is "tight control" of diabetes? Goals, limitations, and evaluation of therapy. Mayo Clin Proc 1986; *61*:792–795.

Soler NG, Frank S: Value of glycosylated hemoglobin measurements after acute myocardial infarction. JAMA 1981; *246*:1690–1693.

Ward WK, Beard JC, Halter JB, et al.: Pathophysiology of insulin secretion in non-insulin-dependent diabetes mellitus. Diabetes Care 1984; *7*:491–502.

Young CW: Rationale for glycemic control. Am J Med 1985; *79*(suppl 3B):8–11.

MONITORING

American Diabetes Association: Bedside blood glucose monitoring in hospitals. Diabetes Care 1986; *9*:89.

American Diabetes Association: Consensus statement on self-monitoring of blood glucose. Diabetes Care 1987; *10*:95–99.

Belsey R, Morrison JI, Whitlow KJ, et al.: Managing bedside glucose testing in the hospital. JAMA 1987; *258*:1634–1638.

Brownlee M, Vlassara H, Cerami A: Nonezymatic glycosylation and the pathogenesis of diabetic complications. Ann Intern Med 1984; *101*:527–537.

Health and Public Policy Committee, American College of Physicians: Glycosylated hemoglobin assays in the management and diagnosis of diabetes mellitus. Ann Intern Med 1984; *101*:710–713.

North DS, Steinzer JF, Woodhouse KM, et al.: Home monitors of blood glucose: Comparison of precision and accuracy. Diabetes Care 1987; *10*:60–66.

Service FJ, O'Brien PC, Rizza RA: Measurements of glucose control. Diabetes Care 1987; *10*:225–237.

COMPLICATIONS

Aaberg T: Advanced diabetic retinopathy: Surgical treatment of complications. Ann Intern Med 1983; *99*:562–563.

Abbott RD, Donahue RP, MacMahon SW, et al.: Diabetes and the risk of stroke: The Honolulu heart program. JAMA 1987; *257*:949–952.

Bending JJ, Viberti GC, Bilous RW, et al.: Eight-month correction of hyperglycemia in insulin-dependent diabetes mellitus is associated with a significant and sustained reduction of urinary albumin excretion rates in patients with microalbuminuria. Diabetes 1985; *34*:69–73.

Ewing DJ, Clarke BF: Diabetic autonomic neuropathy: Present insights and future prospects. Diabetes Care 1986; *9*:648–665.

Greene DA, Lattimer SA, Sima AAF: Sorbitol, phosphoinositides, and sodium-potassium-ATPase in the pathogenesis of diabetic complications. N Engl J Med 1987; *316*:599–606.

Harati Y: Diabetic peripheral neuropathies. Ann Intern Med 1987; *107*:546–559.

Hostetter RH: Diabetic nephropathy. N Engl J Med 1985; *312*:642–644.

Klein R, Moss SE, Klein BEK: New management concepts for timely diagnosis of diabetic retinopathy treatable by photocoagulation. Diabetes Care 1987; *10*:633–638.

Knuiman MW, Welborn TA, McCann VJ, et al.: Prevalence of diabetic complications in relation to risk factors. Diabetes 1986; *35*:1332–1339.

Mogensen CE, Christensen CK: Predicting diabetic nephropathy in insulin-dependent patients. N Engl J Med 1984; *311*:89–93.

Nathan DM, Singer DE, Godine JE, et al.: Non-insulin-dependent diabetes in older patients: Complications and risk factors. Am J Med 1986; *81*:837–842.

Niakan E, Harati Y, Rolak LA, et al.: Silent myocardial infarction and diabetic cardiovascular autonomic neuropathy. Arch Intern Med 1986; *146*:2229–2230.

Oswald GA, Corcoran S, Yudkin JS: Prevalence and risks of hyperglycaemia and undiagnosed diabetes in patients with acute myocardial infarction. Lancet 1984; *1*:1264–1267.

Pulsinelli WA, Levy DE, Sigsbee B, et al.: Increased damage after ischemic stroke in patients with hyperglycemia with or without established diabetes mellitus. Am J Med 1983; *74*:540–543.

Raskin P, Rosenstock J: Aldose reductase inhibitors and diabetic complications. Am J Med 1987; *83*:298–306.

Raskin P, Rosenstock J: Blood glucose control and diabetic complications. Ann Intern Med 1986; *105*:254–263.

Rosenstock J, Raskin P: Early diabetic nephropathy: Assessment and potential therapeutic interventions. Diabetes Care 1986; *9*:529–545.

Rytter L, Troelsen S, Beck-Nielsen H: Prevalence and mortality of acute myocardial infarction in patients with diabetes. Diabetes Care 1985; *8*:230–234.

Winegrad AI: Does a common mechanism induce the diverse complications of diabetes. Diabetes 1987; *36*:396–406.

Zimmerman BR: Current status of aldose reductase inhibitors. Diabetes Care 1987; *10*:123–125.

DIABETIC EMERGENCIES

Khardori R, Soler NG: Hyperosmolar hyperglycemia nonketotic syndrome: Report of 22 cases and brief review. Am J Med 1984; *77*:899–904.

Wachtel TJ, Silliman RA, Lamberton P: Predisposing factors for the diabetic hyperosmolar state. Arch Intern Med 1987; *147*:499–501.

TREATMENT

American Diabetes Association: Nutritional recommendations and principles for individuals with diabetes mellitus: 1986. Diabetes Care 1987; *10*:126–132.

Binder C, Lauritzen T, Faber O, et al.: Insulin pharmacokinetics. Diabetes Care 1984; *7*:188–199.

Clements RS, Bell DSH, Benbarka A, et al.: Rapid insulin initiation in non-insulin-dependent diabetes mellitus. Am J Med 1987; *82*:415–420.

Hoekstra JBL, VanRijn HJM, Thijssen JHH, et al.: C-peptide reactivity as a measure of insulin dependency in obese diabetic patients treated with insulin. Diabetes Care 1982; *5*:585–591.

Martin DB: Type II diabetes: Insulin versus oral agents. N Engl J Med 1986; *314*:1314–1315.

Nathan DM, Roussell A, Godine JE: Glyburide or insulin for metabolic control in non-insulin-dependent diabetes mellitus. Ann Intern Med 1988; *108*:334–340.

National Institutes of Health: Consensus development conference on diet and exercise in non-insulin-dependent diabetes mellitus. Diabetes Care 1987; *10*:639–644.

Kriesberg RA: The second generation sulfonylureas: Change or progress. Ann Intern Med 1985; *102*:125–126.

Raskin P: The Somogyi phenomenon: Sacred cow or bull. Arch Intern Med 1984; *144*:781–787.

Richter EA, Ruderman NB, Schneider SH: Diabetes and exercise. Am J Med 1981; *70*:201–209.

Rizza RA, Gerich JE, Haymond MW, et al.: Control of blood sugar in insulin-dependent diabetes: Comparison of an artificial endocrine pancreas, continuous subcutaneous insulin infusion, and intensified conventional insulin therapy. N Engl J Med 1980; *303*:1313–1318.

Spanheimer RG, DiGirolamo M, Watts NB, et al.: Glycemic response to weight loss in obese diabetic patients. Diabetes 1986; *35*(suppl 1):46a.(Abstract)

Watts NB, Gebhart SSP, Clark RV, et al.: Postoperative management of diabetes mellitus: steady-state glucose control with bedside algorithm for insulin adjustment. Diabetes Care 1987; *10*:722–727.

Wilson RM, Clarke P, Barkes H, et al.: Starting insulin treatment as an outpatient: Report of 100 consecutive patients followed up for at least one year. JAMA 1986; *256*:877–880.

Wing RR, Koeske R, Epstein LH, et al.: Long-term effects of modest weight loss in type II diabetic patients. Arch Intern Med 1987; *147*:1749–1753.

Zimmerman BR: Practical aspects of intensive insulin therapy. Mayo Clin Proc 1986; *61*:806–812.

HYPOGLYCEMIA

Background, Pathophysiology

The body protects itself against low blood glucose through a variety of mechanisms including dietary intake of food, counterregulatory hormones such as epinephrine and glucagon that raise blood glucose acutely, and alternative energy sources such as free fatty acids and ketone bodies. However, when these mechanisms are deranged or inadequate, the result is a drop in blood glucose.

Hypoglycemia means low blood glucose. A difficult question to answer is: "How low is abnormal?" Figure 9–2 shows results of a study by Merimee and Tyson (N Engl J Med 1974; *291*:1275–1278) in which men and women fasted for 72 hours. The lowest glucose value seen in males was 55 mg/dL, but many women had values that were much lower; a few premenopausal women had plasma glucose values between 30 and 40 mg/dL without symptoms and no evidence of underlying disease. Although most physicians would agree that a glucose value <50 mg/dL after an overnight fast indicates the need for further testing, this evidence suggests that glucose levels after a prolonged fast may be lower than most people think.

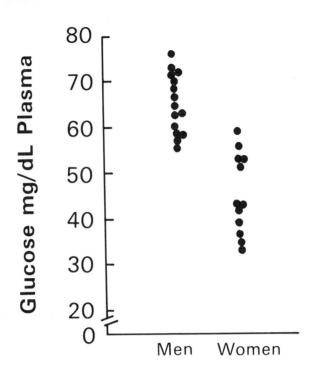

Fig. 9–2. Glucose levels during 72-hour fast, lowest values. (From Merrimee TJ, Tyson J. Reprinted by permission of N Engl J Med 1974; 291:1276.)

Fasting hypoglycemia in adults may be seen with several conditions (Table 9–9). Medications that may cause hypoglycemia include ethanol, sulfonylureas (oral hypoglycemic agents), insulin, and others. Severe liver disease, malnutrition, adrenal insufficiency, and septicemia have all been reported to cause fasting hypoglycemia, but history or physical examination usually point to these causes. Nonendocrine tumors that cause hypoglycemia are usually large mesenchymal tumors that are readily apparent. When these conditions can be excluded,

Table 9–9. Causes of Fasting Hypoglycemia in Adults

Medications (insulin, oral hypoglycemic agents, alcohol, others)
Severe hepatic dysfunction
Glucocorticoid deficiency
Extrapancreatic neoplasms
Hyperinsulinism (insulinoma, islet-cell hyperplasia, nesidioblastosis)

adults who have fasting hypoglycemia usually are found to have an abnormality of insulin secretion or action. Rarely, a circulating antibody binds insulin or an antibody binds with the insulin receptor in target tissues. Most commonly an inappropriate increase in insulin secretion is the cause of fasting hypoglycemia, due either to a tumor of the beta cells producing insulin (called an insulinoma), hyperplasia of the beta cells within the pancreatic islets, or a condition called nesidioblastosis, in which insulin-producing cells proliferate throughout the body of the exocrine pancreas.

After ingestion of a meal, glucose levels first rise, then drop below baseline before stabilizing. The magnitude of the postprandial glucose fall is not well defined but values below 60 mg/dL are not uncommon. A rapid drop in blood glucose usually leads to release of epinephrine and other counterregulatory hormones. Epinephrine produces readily recognizable signs and symptoms such as tachycardia, palpitations, tremor, nervousness, sweating, nausea or hunger, weakness, and fatigue, etc. These adrenergic symptoms occur commonly and are not specific for hypoglycemia, occurring in a variety of other states including hyperthyroidism, pheochromocytoma, and anxiety. When they are triggered by a postprandial fall in serum glucose, it is called reactive hypoglycemia. While this occurs fairly often in patients who have had gastrointestinal surgery, it is uncommon in other situations.

Clinical Presentation

Signs and symptoms that are usually thought of in association with hypoglycemia are the adrenergic manifestations: hunger, palpitations, sweating, dizziness, tremor, and fatigue. In fact, these are not due to hypoglycemia per se but to the release of epinephrine, which in turn is related to the rate of glucose fall.

When blood glucose reaches a low level, usually less than 40 mg/dL, function of the central nervous system is affected. This is called *neuroglycopenia.* Symptoms and signs of neuroglycopenia include confusion, lethargy, coma, and convulsions. If the rate of glucose fall is gradual, neuroglycopenia may occur without premonitory adrenergic symptoms. Table 9–10 contrasts neuroglycopenic with adrenergic symptoms.

Diagnosis of Hypoglycemia

Hypoglycemia has been a widely diagnosed condition for years. There are many reasons to believe that this diagnosis is often made in error. The American Diabetes Association (Dia-

Table 9–10. Symptoms and Signs of Hypoglycemia

ADRENERGIC
  hunger, palpitations, sweating
  dizziness, tremor, fatigue
    related to rate of glucose fall
    due to release of epinephrine

NEUROGLYCOPENIC
  confusion, lethargy, coma, convulsions
  affects central nervous system

NOTE: Adrenergic symptoms occur commonly, and are not specific for hypoglycemia

betes Care 1982; 5:72) issued this statement: "The majority of people with these kinds of (adrenergic) symptoms do not have hypoglycemia; a great many patients with anxiety reactions present with similar symptoms. Furthermore, there is no good evidence that hypoglycemia causes depression, chronic fatigue, allergies, nervous breakdowns, alcoholism, juvenile delinquency, childhood behavior problems, drug addiction, or inadequate sexual performance."

Many people experience adrenergic symptoms 2 or 3 hours after meals and find that eating relieves their symptoms. Many of these same people have similar symptoms 2 to 4 hours after an oral glucose load, at a time when their blood glucose is below 60 mg/dL. However, most of these people will *not* have low blood glucose at the times their symptoms occur in daily life or after a test meal. Also, as many as 25% of healthy subjects will have glucose values under 60 mg/dL during an oral glucose tolerance test. It seems unwise to assign a "disease" to 25% of the population based only on GTT results.

In subjects with adrenergic symptoms after eating, something is different from usual. The symptoms cannot be ascribed to hypoglycemia, since they occur when blood glucose level is normal. The symptoms are probably related to some aspect of digestion or gastrointestinal hormones. The precise mechanism of this disorder is not clear. What is clear is the confusion in the diagnosis of reactive hypoglycemia, and that a 4-, 5- or 6-hour oral glucose tolerance test does not appear to aid in diagnosis or management. Several investigators have suggested referring to this condition as the idiopathic postprandial syndrome. Anxiety (such as fear of potentially serious medical problems) aggravates this condition. Most of these patients improve when they are reassured that their condition is not going to change into something worse.

To exclude the diagnosis of reactive hypoglycemia (or to confirm it in the rare patient when it truly occurs), it is best to *avoid doing a glucose tolerance test.* The circumstances of the OGTT are artificial. Dietary carbohydrate restriction causes "reactive" hypoglycemia on OGTT that is reversible after carbohydrate loading. If the patient has frequent symptomatic episodes, it may be possible to document a normal venous plasma glucose during symptoms. If episodes are infrequent, most patients can be trained to do capillary self blood glucose testing during symptoms. Finally, a meal tolerance test can be done (protocol, p. 216), with a standard breakfast replacing the oral glucose load of a 5-hour GTT. All these strategies are designed to establish for the physician and the patient that blood glucose is *not* low when symptoms occur.

True hypoglycemia is an infrequent cause of disease, but when it does occur, it is usually serious. The symptoms associated with *fasting hypoglycemia* may be adrenergic or neuroglycopenic or both. Hypoglycemia and symptoms usually occur in the fasting state, but may also occur after meals. Hypoglycemic symptoms are usually relieved within 15 to 20 mintues of eating. Whipple's triad provides the classic criteria for the diagnosis of organic hypoglycemia. These criteria include: (1) symptoms of hypoglycemia (either adrenergic or neuroglycopenic), (2) documentation that blood glucose is low during symptoms, and (3) relief of symptoms with glucose or food.

When fasting hypoglycemia is suspected, it is advisable to admit the patient to the hospital for a supervised period of fasting. Serum or plasma glucose should be measured by the laboratory every 4 hours and any time the patient is symptomatic (reflectance meters are not sufficiently accurate to use for this purpose). Most patients with endogenous hyperinsulinism will become hypoglycemic under fasting conditions; 35% will become hypoglycemic in 12 hours or less, 75% in 24 hours, and over 90% will be hypoglycemic in 48 hours. When hypoglycemia occurs (glucose <60 mg/dL), measurement of plasma insulin and C-peptide in simultaneous sample will show inappropriately elevated values in most patients with insulinoma.

Several formulas have been suggested for expressing insulin and glucose levels in these patients, with hopes of improving diagnostic accuracy. Figure 9–3 shows work from Service and colleagues (Mayo Clin Proc 1976; *51*:417–429); each dot represents a patient with a proven insulinoma, with the patient's plasma glucose shown on the horizontal axis and plasma insulin on the vertical axis. The lines across the chart represent

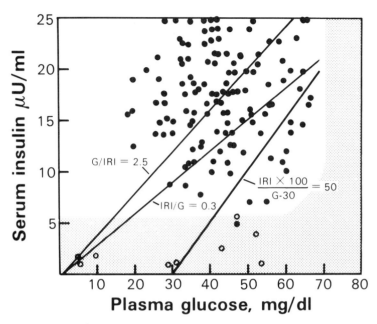

Fig. 9–3. Simultaneous serum insulin and plasma glucose in patients with proven insulinoma (closed circles) and noninsulin-mediated hypoglycemia (open circles). The lines indicate various ratios used to diagnose insulinoma; for each ratio, closed circles to the right of the line would be classified as false negative by that ratio. (Used with permission from Service FJ: Hypoglycemic Disorders. Boston, GK Hall Medical Publishers, 1983. By permission of Mayo Foundation.)

three suggested formulas for expressing the data. Each dot to the right of a line is a patient with an insulinoma who would have been classified as normal by that formula. Based on this analysis, Dr. Service recommends making the diagnosis of insulinoma based on an inappropriately elevated serum insulin, over 6 μU/mL, at a time the plasma glucose is under 60 mg/dL. This requires a precise and sensitive assay for insulin.

Insulin and C-peptide are both elevated in most patients with insulinoma. Even if insulin levels are quite high, C-peptide measurement is a helpful confirmatory finding; occasionally, C-peptide is elevated when insulin is normal. Measurement of C-peptide is invaluable to resolve the suspicion of surreptitious injection of insulin as a cause for hypoglycemia; if exogenous insulin is administered, C-peptide is low when serum insulin is high. Proinsulin measurement is technically difficult and usually unnecessary in the evaluation of suspected hyperinsulinism. Under normal circumstances, only a small amount of proinsulin is released into the circulation. Proinsulin has much less biologic activity than insulin, but large amounts may cause hypoglycemia. Occasional cases of insulinoma have been reported in which insulin and C-peptide values were normal but proinsulin was strikingly elevated.

Once biochemical evidence of inappropriate hyperinsulinism is found, *localization studies* should be performed. CT or MR of the pancreas will show many of these tumors. Transhepatic transportal pancreatic vein sampling for insulin measurement may also be done. There is no substitute for a skilled and experienced surgeon for proper localization.

Treatment

Alimentary hypoglycemia after gastric surgery can often be managed by diet (small, frequent feedings and avoidance of sugar and sweets). Pharmacologic measures, if necessary, include anticholinergics to slow gastric emptying or beta-adrenergic blocking agents to blunt the symptoms. In intractable cases, surgery such as interposition of an antiperistaltic jejunal segment may be required to slow gastric emptying. The same dietary and pharmacologic measures may be used in patients with reactive hypoglycemia in the absence of gastrointestinal surgery and in patients with idiopathic postprandial syndrome. Not yet available for general use are agents such as acarbose that block digestion and absorption of starches, which may be of some help in this problem.

Patients with hyperinsulinism are best treated by surgical removal of the tumor or, if the problem is beta cell-hyperplasia or nesidioblastosis, by subtotal pancreatectomy. Persistent hypoglycemia may be improved with diazoxide (Proglycem), 3 to 8 mg/kg/day in divided doses, but side effects of fluid retention and hirsutism limit its use. Long-acting analogs of somatostatin have recently become available and may offer better medical treatment. Malignant insulinomas may respond to chemotherapy with conventional agents or streptozotocin.

Chandalia HB, Boshell BR: Hypoglycemia associated with extrapancreatic tumors. Arch Intern Med 1979; *129*:447–456.

Charles MA, Hofeldt F, Shackelford A, et al.: Comparison of oral glucose tolerance tests and mixed meals in patients with apparent postabsorptive hypoglycemia: absence of hypoglycemia after meals. Diabetes 1981; *30*:465–470.

Gastineau CF: Is reactive hypoglycemia a clinical entity? Mayo Clin Proc 1983; *58*:545–549.

Grunberger G, Weiner JL, Silverman R, et al.: Factitious hypoglycemia due to surreptitious administration of insulin: Diagnosis, treatment, and long-term follow up. Ann Intern Med 1988; *108*:252–257.

Hogan MJ, Service FJ, Sharborough FW, et al.: Oral glucose tolerance test compared with a mixed meal in the diagnosis of reactive hypoglycemia: a caveat on stimulation. Mayo Clin Proc 1983; *58*:491–496.

Merimee TJ, Tyson JE: Stabilization of plasma glucose during fasting. N Engl J Med 1974; *291*:1275–1278.

Nelson RL: Hypoglycemia: fact or fiction? Mayo Clin Proc 1985; *60*:844–850.

Permutt MA, Delmez J, Stenson W: Effects of carbohydrate restriction on the hypoglycemic phase of the glucose tolerance test. J Clin Endocrinol Metab 1976; *43*:1088–1093.

Rizza RA, Gerich JE: Statement on hypoglycemia. Diabetes Care 1982; *5*:72–73.

Seltzer HS: Drug-induced hypoglycemia. Diabetes 1972; *21*:955–964.

Service FJ: Hypoglycemia Disorders: Pathogenesis, Diagnosis, and Treatment. Boston, GK Hall Medical Publishers, 1983.

Service FJ, Dale AJD, Elveback LR, et al.: Insulinoma. Mayo Clin Proc 1976; *51*:417–429.

Watts NB: Oral glucose tolerance test may be done too fast. Lab World 1981; *32*:68–72.

10

Lipids and Lipoproteins

LIPIDS AND LIPOPROTEINS

Background, Pathophysiology

There are two basic types of lipids in blood: cholesterol and triglycerides. These lipids are carried in the circulation bound to carrier proteins known as *lipoproteins.* The handling of lipoproteins is controlled by enzymes and specific apoproteins.

Figure 10–1 shows the pathways of lipid absorption, metabolism, and excretion. After absorption, dietary fats are transported via lymphatics as *chylomicrons.* Upon reaching the circulation, chylomicrons are catabolized by the enzyme *lipoprotein lipase* (LPL) to *chylomicron remnants,* which are cleared by the liver. The liver produces *very low-density lipoproteins* (VLDL), which are also cleared by lipoprotein lipase. The lipid that is not stored in adipose tissue is converted to smaller particles, *intermediate-density lipoproteins* (IDL) and *low-density lipoproteins* (LDL). LDL and IDL are taken up by peripheral tissues and the liver by cell surface LDL-receptors. *High-density lipoproteins* (HDL) are formed in the liver and intestine and aid in the catabolism of LDL and in the transport of lipid to the liver for excretion in bile.

Apoproteins are specific compounds associated with lipoprotein structure and metabolism. In structure, apoprotein A1 is the major constituent of HDL lipoprotein; apo-B100 is present in VLDL and is the sole protein component of LDL. Apoproteins serve as cofactors for enzymes involved in lipoprotein metabolism: apo-C1 and C2 for lipoprotein lipase (LPL) and apo-A1 for lecithin-cholesterol acyl transferase (LCAT), apo-B100 interacts with the LDL receptor, apo-E is involved in chylomicron removal, and apo-A1 interacts with the HDL receptor.

Levels of lipids and lipoproteins are determined by diet and physical conditioning, as well as acquired and inherited disorders of lipid metabolism.

Hypercholesterolemia, whether due to diet or a specific lip-

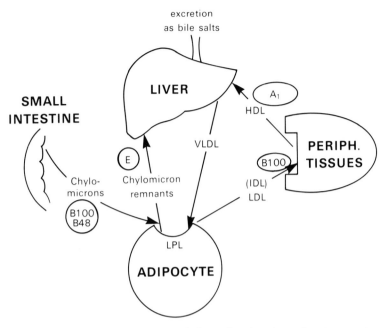

Fig. 10–1. Metabolic pathways of cholesterol and triglycerides. Apoprotein interactions are shown in circles. Abbreviations: HDL, high density lipoproteins; IDL, intermediate density lipoproteins; LDL, low density lipoproteins; LPL, lipoprotein lipase; VLDL, very low density lipoproteins.

oprotein disorder, has been recognized as one of several important risk factors for cardiovascular disease. Levels of cholesterol (particularly the highly atherogenic LDL fraction) in the United States population are high compared to most other countries. Atherosclerosis is associated with high LDL cholesterol and low HDL cholesterol, or both. The main reason for identification is the reduction of the potential for atherosclerosis through dietary changes or medication.

Levels of triglycerides (high VLDL) above 500 mg/dL are associated with an increased risk for pancreatitis. The association of triglycerides with atherosclerosis is not clear or strong (with the exception of primary type III hyperlipoproteinemia, which is rare).

Table 10–1 shows the lipid and protein composition of the major classes of lipoproteins and their relative atherogenicity. Table 10–2 shows a practical clinical classification based on measurements of cholesterol and triglycerides. The Fredrickson classification (phenotypes I, II, III, IV, and V) is of historical

Table 10–1. Constituents and Clinical Implications of Major Circulating Lipid Fractions

Lipoprotein	Major Lipid	Apoproteins	Atherogenicity
Chylomicrons	Triglycerides	C2	None
Chylo. remnants and IDL	Triglycerides (50%) Cholesterol (50%)	C1,C2,C3,E	Yes
VLDL	Triglycerides (80%) Cholesterol (20%)	C3,B100,E	Possible
LDL	Cholesterol	B100	High
HDL	Cholesterol	A1	Protective

Table 10–2. Clinical Classification of Primary Disorders of Lipoprotein Metabolism

Elevated Plasma Lipid	Elevated Lipoprotein	Lipoprotein Phenotype
Triglycerides only	chylomicrons	type I
	chylos + VLDL	type V
	VLDL only	type IV
Cholesterol only	LDL	type IIa
Cholesterol and triglycerides	LDL + VLDL	type IIb
	IDL	type III

(From Hoeg JM, Gregg RE, Brewer HB Jr: An approach to the management of hyperlipoproteinemia. JAMA 1986; *255*:512–521.)

interest. However, description by specific lipids and lipoprotein fractions should be encouraged.

Secondary causes of hyperlipoproteinemias should be considered in the differential diagnosis and include hypothyroidism, nephrotic syndrome, and multiple myeloma.

Clinical Presentation

The detection of most lipoprotein disorders is made in the laboratory. Rarely, patients with lipid disorders have physical signs (lipemia retinalis, eruptive or tendinous xanthomas). Lipid deposits around the eyelids (xanthelasma) or iris (arcus senilis or arcus corneae) do not correlate with serum lipid levels. Symptoms are usually absent unless due to associated conditions (atherosclerosis, pancreatitis).

Diagnosis

The main reason for diagnosing lipid disorders is to identify persons at high risk for atherosclerosis because of the lipid abnormality, then reduce the undesirable lipid class with diet or medication, hoping to reduce the later development of ath-

189

erosclerosis. There is increasing evidence that this line of reasoning is correct, but still disagreement over who should be tested (screening everyone or only patients with other risk factors), how to test (measure total cholesterol, calculate LDL cholesterol, or measure apoproteins), and how to best treat specific lipid abnormalities.

The clinical importance of cholesterol and its subfractions is still being debated. The decision to treat for a cholesterol abnormality should not be made on the laboratory result alone, but with full consideration to the patient's other coronary risk factors. The National Cholesterol Education Program has proposed the following limits: for total cholesterol, desirable is below 200 mg/dL and elevated is above 240 mg/dL; for LDL cholesterol, desirable is below 130 mg/dL and elevated is above 160 mg/dL. Treatment, initially with diet, then medication if diet is not effective, is recommended for all patients with elevated levels and for patients with borderline levels who have two or more cardiac risk factors (e.g., cigarette smoking, diabetes mellitus, obesity, family history of premature cardiovascular disease) (Table 10–3).

Since atherogenicity is associated with the LDL cholesterol subfraction, decisions for treatment are best based on LDL levels rather than total cholesterol. A logical approach to initial testing is to use total cholesterol, preferably but not necessarily on a fasting blood sample. If total cholesterol is below 200 mg/dL (or below 240 mg/dL in someone with no other cardiovascular risk factors), no additional testing would be needed, though repeat testing 1 to 5 years later should be done. If total cholesterol is above 240 mg/dL (or above 200 mg/dL in someone with two or more cardiac risk factors), cholesterol subfractions should be determined. This should be done only on a fasting blood sample. Before making a final decision regarding treatment, samples from several different days should be obtained to establish a baseline.

Table 10–3.   Decision Levels for Hypercholesterolemia

	Total Cholesterol (mg/dL)	LDL Cholesterol (mg/dL)	Treatment*
Desirable	<200	<130	No
Borderline	200–240	130–160	If cardiac risk factors are present
Elevated	>240	>160	All patients

*Treatment should be with diet initially, then with medication if diet is not fully effective.

To determine cholesterol subfractions, measurements of total cholesterol, HDL cholesterol, and triglycerides are performed. LDL is calculated from these values using the following formula, which is valid as long as triglycerides are below 500 mg/dL:

$$LDL = \text{total cholesterol} - HDL - (\text{triglycerides}/5).$$

The narrow range of cholesterol levels recommended for intervention demands a high degree of laboratory precision and accuracy. This can be achieved by the use of standard reference materials that are now available. Not all methods for measurement of cholesterol give satisfactory results. Before using cholesterol results for diagnosis or for follow-up of treatment, the performance of the laboratory being used should be known.

There is good correlation between the presence of atherosclerosis and apoprotein levels, a ratio of apo-A to apo-B below 1.325 indicating a high risk. Whether this information adds to the value of determination of cholesterol subfractions in the average patient is not clear.

Treatment

Dietary modification should be considered for almost all patients with lipoprotein disorders. If the patient is obese, calories should be reduced to reach and maintain a desirable body weight. Limiting cholesterol intake to 300 mg daily and increasing mono- and polyunsaturated fats is advisable; the "prudent diet" of the American Heart Association provides a good general guide. Increasing dietary fiber may be useful. Improved physical conditioning is advisable. LDL levels are increased by commonly used antihypertensive agents, thiazide diuretics and beta-adrenergic blocking drugs; these agents should be used with caution (if at all) in patients known to have hyperlipidemia. Patients with high VLDL or IDL should abstain from alcohol. If dietary measures fail to lower lipid levels sufficiently, pharmacologic treatment should be considered.

The ideal end point of lipid-lowering therapy is still being debated. While the NIH Consensus Development Conference recommended lowering total serum cholesterol below 200 mg/dL, lesser decreases may be of substantial benefit to some individuals. It has been shown that a 1% reduction in total cholesterol results in a 2% decrease in cardiovascular risk.

Niacin would seem an ideal drug for treatment of patients with most forms of hyperlipidemia; it is inexpensive and it has beneficial effects on all classes of atherogenic lipoproteins, raising HDL cholesterol but lowering LDL cholesterol and VLDL triglycerides. Intolerance to the drug limits its use; therapeutic doses cause uncomfortable cutaneous flushing in almost all patients, and many patients experience severe gastrointestinal side effects. Acceptance can be increased by beginning with a low dose of the drug (100 mg tid), gradually working up to a maximum dose of 2 g tid; giving the drug with meals but not with hot beverages; and giving aspirin an hour before the dose if flushing is severe. Warning the patient about these potential side effects is important. Liver chemistries, glucose, and uric acid levels must be monitored periodically.

Agents or measures that *increase HDL cholesterol* include, exercise, increased lean body mass, moderate ethanol ingestion, estrogens (in females), and niacin.

Agents that *reduce VLDL levels,* in addition to niacin, include the fibric acid derivatives clofibrate, gemfibrozil, and probucol. However, some studies indicate that use of these agents may be associated with increased cardiovascular mortality. Hepatotoxicity may occur, so liver chemistries should be checked periodically. Since increased VLDL is not clearly associated with increased cardiovascular mortality, a decision to use one of these agents should not be made lightly. Gemfibrozil may be useful in some patients with elevated LDL cholesterol and has been shown in the Helsinki Heart Study to reduce the risk of coronary artery disease with no increase in other mortality.

Agents that *reduce LDL cholesterol,* in addition to niacin, include the bile acid sequestrants cholestyramine (Questran) and colestipol (Colestid). Constipation is almost universal with these agents; patients should be warned of this and advised to use a stool softener if needed. The taste can be improved by refrigeration. Best tolerance is achieved by beginning with a low dose and gradually increasing to full levels. These agents may cause increases in VLDL, so triglycerides should be monitored. The possibility that these agents may interfere with the absorption of other medications must be kept in mind. If bile acid sequestrants are not fully effective or are not tolerated, clofibrate or gemfibrozil may be tried; however, these drugs are of limited effectiveness for lowering LDL cholesterol.

Lovastatin (Mevacor), an agent recently approved for use in this country, shows great promise for lowering LDL cholesterol. It appears to work by blocking intracellular synthesis of cholesterol through inhibition of the intracellular enzyme HMG-CoA reductase. This results in an increase in cell surface LDL receptors. In clinical trials it appears effective and well tolerated. Regular eye examinations and liver chemistries are recommended to monitor side effects. If safety can be established, cost can be reduced, and the good experience with this agent holds up with more widespread use, this drug will likely become the first line of pharmacologic treatment for patients with elevated LDL cholesterol.

The Expert Panel: Report of the National Cholesterol Education Program on Detection, Evaluation, and Treatment of High Blood Cholesterol in Adults. Arch Intern Med 1988; *148*:36–69.

Fihn SD: A prudent approach to control of cholesterol levels. JAMA 1987; *258*:2416–2418.

Gordon DJ, Rifkind BM: 3-Hydroxy-3-methylglutaryl coenzyme A (HMG-CoA) reductase inhibitors: a new class of cholesterol-lowering agents. Ann Intern Med 1987; *107*:759–761.

Grundy MS: Cholesterol and coronary heart disease: A new era. JAMA 1986; *256*:2849–2858.

Havel RJ, Hunninghake DM, Illingworth DR, et al.: Lovastatin (mevinolin) in the treatment of heterozygous familial hypercholesterolemia. Ann Intern Med 1987; *107*:609–615.

Hoeg JM, Gregg RE, Brewer HB Jr: An approach to the management of hyperlipoproteinemia. JAMA 1986; *255*:512–521.

Kuske TT, Feldman EB: Hyperlipoproteinemia, atherosclerosis risk, and dietary management. Arch Intern Med 1987; *147*:357–360.

Leaf A, Weber PC: Cardiovascular effects of n-3 fatty acids. N Engl J Med 1988; *318*:549–557.

Palumbo PJ: National cholesterol education program: Does the emperor have any clothes? Mayo Clin Proc 1988; *63*:88–90.

Rifkind BM: Gemfibrozil, lipids, and coronary risk. N Engl J Med 1987; *317*:1279–1281.

Schaefer EJ, Levey RI: Pathogenesis and management of lipoprotein disorders. N Engl J Med 1985; *312*:1300–1310.

Sullivan JM, Vader Zwaag R, Lemp GF, et al.: Postmenopausal estrogen use and coronary atherosclerosis. Ann Intern Med 1988; *108*:358–363.

Von Schacky C: Prophylaxis of atherosclerosis with marine omega-3 fatty acids: A comprehensive strategy. Ann Intern Med 1987; *107*:890–899.

11

Miscellaneous Topics

OBESITY

Obesity is an excess of adipose tissue, the result of ingestion and absorption of more calories than needed to satisfy metabolic requirements. Ideally, there is balance between caloric intake and metabolic demands that results in a stable, "ideal" weight. If metabolic demands are reduced, a reduction in calorie intake should maintain this balance. If metabolic demands are reduced but weight is gained, there must be a defect in this balance, possibly in the hypothalamic centers for satiety or hunger. There appear to be many factors that contribute to obesity.

One factor may be the number of fat cells. Weight gain in childhood is associated with an increase in the number of adipose cells. Since cell number cannot be reduced, weight reduction results in a subnormal content of lipid per cell. Weight gain in adults causes an increase in the fat content of adipose cells with no change in the number of cells, so, at least in theory, weight reduction can occur without dropping the fat content of cells below normal. None of this evidence explains why obesity develops—why caloric intake is not reduced when needs are less.

It is unusual to be able to identify a specific cause of obesity. Obesity often occurs in states of excess cortisol or insulin, or deficient thyroid hormone, but these conditions are usually suspected on clinical grounds. When using laboratory tests to look for underlying metabolic disorders or disease states in obesity, the physician should be thoughtful and selective. If thyroid or adrenal dysfunction is suspected, tests may be ordered as outlined in the respective chapters. The association of obesity with disorders such as the polycystic ovary syndrome suggests a causal relationship, but the mechanism is unclear. Finding obesity with a strong family preponderance or in rare genetic disorders such as Prader-Willi syndrome suggests that inherited factors are important. Environmental factors such as social patterns of eating and drinking and cultural standards for desirable weights can be important in determining the prevalence of obesity.

Obesity predisposes to diabetes mellitus, gout, and menstrual disturbance as secondary conditions. There may be an association between the distribution of obesity (central vs lower segment, or "apple" vs "pear") and these secondary conditions. Mortality is somewhat higher in obese people than persons of "desirable" weight.

As with many conditions, the evaluation of the patient with obesity should begin with a history and physical examination. Desirable weights for age and sex may be found in life insurance tables or roughly estimated using the Hamwi formula, which for males assigns 106 pounds for the first 5 feet of height and 6 pounds for each additional inch; for females, 100 pounds for the first 5 feet and 5 pounds for each additional inch. For example, if a man is 5'10" tall, 106 pounds plus (6 pounds × 10 inches) = 106 + 66 = 172 pounds. If a woman is 5'4" tall, 100 pounds plus (5 pounds × 4 inches) = 100 + 20 = 120 pounds. These calculations are only estimates, with a potential error of at least 10%.

The problem of obesity remains one without simple explanations or solutions. Although obesity is a concomitant of various endocrine disorders (hypothyroidism, Cushing's syndrome), obesity is rarely due to identifiable factors. Evaluation should include TSH or other tests to exclude hypothyroidism, and urine free cortisol in patients with features in addition to obesity that suggest Cushing's syndrome. Treatment of obesity requires patience and flexibility. The goals of treatment should include not only weight loss, but prevention of regain or additional gain.

Rather than prescribing a "diet," helping the patient with changes in eating habits should be effective in meeting these goals. Programs that emphasize sound nutrition and behavior modification are available in most areas. "Fad" diets and programs that emphasize quick weight loss are rarely effective in the long run.

For moderate obesity, life-style changes should be recommended: modest calorie restriction and regular physical activity. For morbid obesity, or moderate obesity complicated by severe medical problems, surgery (reducing gastric capacity) or an intragastric balloon may be considered.

Medical treatment of obesity does not offer much. Amphetamine-related appetite suppressant medication may be of short term use in a few specific instances (e.g., an obese patient who requires an elective abdominal operation and short-term weight loss may be of benefit). Efforts are underway to develop medication that will interfere with the absorption of food, allowing the luxury of eating food simply for the pleasure of eating, without having to deal with the calories later.

Bray GA (ed): Obesity in America. NIH publication no. 79–359, Bethesda, National Institutes of Health, 1979.

Health implications of obesity: National Institutes of Health Consensus Development Conference statement. Ann Intern Med 1985; *103*:147–151.

Moss JA: Caution: Very-low-calorie diets can be deadly. Ann Intern Med 1985; *102*:121–123.

Newmark SR, Williamson B: Survey of very-low-calorie weight reduction diets: I. Novelty diets. Arch Intern Med 1983; *143*:1195–1198.

Newmark SR, Williamson B:Survey of very-low-calorie weight reduction diets: II. Total fasting, protein sparing modified fasts, chemically defined diets. Arch Intern Med 1983; *143*:1423–1427.

Rosenberg IH: Starch blockers—still no calorie-free lunch. N Engl J Med 1982; *307*:1444-1445.

Sparrow D, Borkan GA, Gerzof SG, et al.: Relationship of fat distribution to glucose tolerance: Results of computed tomography in male participants of normative aging study. Diabetes 1986; *35*:411–415.

Van Itallie TB, Kral JG: The dilemma of morbid obesity. JAMA 1981; *246*:999–1003.

ECTOPIC HORMONES AND PARANEOPLASTIC SYNDROMES

Background, Pathophysiology

Malignant neoplasms may produce a variety of products that cause striking clinical effects. These products are termed ectopic when they are not normally derived from the tissue of origin of the tumor. The potential for neoplasms to produce hormones ectopically is due in part to the derivation of many tumors from neural ectoderm, small cells that have amine precursor uptake and decarboyxlase activity (APUD cells). Although not all hormone-producing malignancies are derived from APUD cells, probably all cancers can produce and secrete one or more proteins or peptides. Not all tumor products are biologically active, and none are specific for a particular cell type. As tumor markers, however, these substances attract great interest.

Hormones are among the markers produced by neoplasms (Table 11–1). In many instances, these markers lack biologic activity, but their measurement may be useful in the diagnosis of certain malignancies or in following the response to treat-

Table 11–1. Ectopic Hormones Produced by Malignant Tumors

ACTH, proACTH	Corticotropin-releasing
Lipotropin	hormone (CRH)
Somatomedins	Calcitonin
Parathyroid hormone	Antidiuretic hormone
Prolactin, "big" prolactin	(vasopressin)
Gastrin	Prostaglandins
Glucagon	Growth hormone
Chorionic somatomammotropin	Secretin
Erythropoetin	Somatostatin
Chorionic gonadotropin (intact	Vasoactive intestinal
and beta-subunit)	polypeptide
Pituitary glycoprotein hormones	
(alpha subunit)	

(Used by permission from Chattoraj SC, Watts NB: *in* Tietz NB (ed): Textbook of Clinical Chemistry, Philadelphia, WB Saunders, 1987, p 1161.)

ment. Some neoplasms may exhibit markers inconsistently, not at all, or variably with the natural progression of the tumor.

Most frequently, the ectopically produced substances are similar to the naturally occurring hormones and are therefore detectable with standard immunoassay techniques. If there are immunochemical differences between the ectopic and natural hormones, they are usually not sufficient for most assays to distinguish normal from ectopic production.

One study suggests that ectopic hormone production, at least for small cell lung tumors, carries a better prognosis than similar tumors without paraneoplastic syndromes.

Clinical Presentation

The most commonly encountered instances of ectopic hormone production are ectopic ACTH associated with oat-cell carcinomas of the lung, bronchial and other carcinoid tumors, and with medullary carcinomas of the thyroid; ectopic ADH (SIADH) associated with oat-cell and other malignancies of the lung, and carcinomas of the ovary. In most cases of humoral hypercalcemia, the exact mediator of hypercalcemia is not yet known; it has many of the actions of parathyroid hormone but is immunochemically quite different. Ectopic production of parathyroid hormone has not been demonstrated. With ectopic production of ACTH, the typical picture of cortisol excess (Cushing's syndrome) is often overshadowed by wasting associated with the tumor.

Diagnosis and Treatment

The diagnosis of ectopic hormone production should be suspected when a tumor is found that is known to be associated with hormone production. The clinician should be aware of the possible hormones involved and look for manifestations (hyponatremia from SIADH, hypokalemia and hyperglycemia from ACTH, or hypercalcemia from humoral substances). Standard approaches to the differential diagnosis of eutopically derived hormone excess should be applied when ectopic hormone production is suspected (e.g., the standard evaluation for Cushing's syndrome for suspected ectopic ACTH). Treatment of the hormone excess states can be determined based on treatment options discussed for the specific hormones.

Abeloff MD: Paraneoplastic syndromes: A window on the biology of cancer. N Engl J Med 1987; *317*:1598–1600.

Baylin SB, Mendelshon G: Ectopic (inappropriate) hormone production by tumors: Mechanisms involved and the biological and clinical implications. Endocrine Rev 1980; *1*:45–77.

Bostwick DG, Null WE, Holmes D, et al.: Expression of opioid peptides in tumors. N Engl J Med 1987; *317*:1439–1443.

Burtis WJ, Wu T, Insogna KL, et al: Humoral hypercalcemia of malignancy. Ann Intern Med 1988; *108*:454–457.

de la Monte AM, Hutchins GM, Moore GW: Paraneoplastic syndromes and constitutional symptoms in prediction of metastatic behavior of small cell carcinoma of the lung. Am J Med 1984; *77*:851–856.

Klee GG, Go VLW: Serum tumor markers. Mayo Clin Proc 1982; *57*:129–132.

Odell WD, Wolfsen RA: Hormones from tumors: Are they ubiquitous? Am J Med 1980; *68*:317–318.

Rosen SW, Weintraub BD: Humors, tumors, and caveats. Ann Intern Med 1975; *82*:274–276.

Weichert RF: The neural ectodermal origin of the peptide-secreting endocrine glands. Am J Med 1970; *49*:232–241.

MULTIPLE ENDOCRINE NEOPLASIA (MEN) SYNDROMES

Neoplasia of multiple endocrine glands is present in at least three distinct syndromes. These are shown in Table 11–2. Types I and IIa are inherited in autosomal dominant fashion; the inheritance of type IIb is probably autosomal dominant but is not well worked out. The reason for the coincidence of tumors of multiple endocrine glands is unclear, but probably relates to the origin from cells of amine precursor uptake and decarboxylase (APUD) origin.

If a person is known to belong to a kindred with one of these syndromes, some sort of testing and periodic surveillance is in

Table 11–2. Features of Multiple Neoplasia Syndromes

Type	Involvement
I (Wermer's syndrome)	Parathyroid Pancreas Pituitary
IIa (Sipple's syndrome)	Medullary carcinoma of the thyroid Pheochromocytoma Parathyroid
IIb	Mucocutaneous neuromas Pheochromocytoma Medullary carcinoma of the thyroid

order. Exactly what to test and how often are questions that do not have simple answers. However, in most patients with endocrine neoplasia involving a single gland (e.g., hyperparathyroidism), the condition is sporadic rather than familial. Of the different tumors involved in MEN syndromes, medullary carcinoma of the thyroid (MCT) is the most likely to be inherited (25% of cases), a fact that merits looking for cases of MCT in other family members and looking for pheochromocytoma in patients with MCT. Sporadic hyperparathyroidism is usually due to a single adenoma, while the hyperparathyroidism of MEN syndromes is due to hyperplasia; thus, patients with parathyroid hyperplasia should be considered as possible MEN candidates, with additional disorders looked for in the patient and family members.

How to best look for the different endocrine tumors is fairly straightforward: serum calcium for hyperparathyroidism, 24-hour urine metanephrine for pheochromocytoma, calcitonin (basal or stimulated with pentagastrin and calcium) for medullary carcinoma of the thyroid. Pituitary tumors associated with MEN-I may be nonsecretory (detected by mass effects on visual fields or sellar enlargement on skull x ray) or produce Cushing's syndrome, acromegaly, or hyperprolactinemia. Diagnosis of pancreatic tumors offers the greatest challenge; tumors producing insulin, gastrin (Zollinger-Ellison syndrome with intractable peptic ulcer disease), vasoactive intestinal polypeptide (Verner-Morrison syndrome with watery diarrhea), glucagon, somatostatin, and pancreatic polypeptide have all been described.

When to test for these tumors in asymptomatic family members is a more important question. In MEN-I, hyperparathyroidism precedes other endocrine neoplasia in almost all cases, so simply following serum calcium at yearly intervals is probably sufficient. Serum gastrin and pancreatic polypeptide seem to be the best markers for pancreatic tumors with MEN, but routine measurement of these hormones is not likely to be cost-effective. Medullary carcinoma of the thyroid is a serious condition but potentially curable if detected early, so testing with calcitonin measurements (basal and stimulated) is warranted in all patients at risk; how often to do these tests is debatable.

Benson L, Ljunghall S, Akerstrom G, et al.: Hyperparathyroidism presenting as the first lesion in multiple endocrine neoplasia type 1. Am J Med 1987; *82*:731–738.

Gogel HK, Buckman MT, Cadieux D, et al.: Gastric secretion and hormonal interactions in multiple endocrine neoplasia type I. Arch Intern Med 1985; *145*:855–859.

Oberg K, Walinder O, Bostrom H, et al.: Peptide hormone markers in screening for endocrine tumors in multiple endocrine adenomatosis type I. Am J Med 1982; *73*:619–630.

Yamaguchi K, Kameya T, Abe K: Multiple endocrine neoplasia type I. Clin Endocrinol Metab 1980; *9*:261–284.

SEROTONIN AND THE CARCINOID SYNDROME

Background, Pathophysiology

Serotonin (5-hydroxytryptamine, 5-HT) is a powerful smooth-muscle stimulant and vasoconstrictor derived from the amino acid tryptophan. It is transported in the blood by platelets. Serotonin is metabolized by the enzyme monoamine oxidase (MAO) to form 5-hydroxyindoleacetic acid (5-HIAA), the most significant metabolite. The most important physiologic function of serotonin is as a neurotransmitter. In humans, serotonin has been implicated in a variety of behavioral patterns including sleep, perception of pain, social behavior, and mental depression.

Carcinoid tumors arise from neuroendocrine cells in locations derived from the embryonic gut. These cells are widely distributed throughout the gastrointestinal tract, biliary tract and gallbladder, pancreatic ducts, and bronchial tree and are also found in the thymus, thyroid, ovary, uterus, and salivary glands. Carcinoid tumors of foregut and midgut origin have the capacity to produce serotonin and the classic *carcinoid syndrome.* Since most carcinoid tumors drain into the portal vein and serotonin is rapidly cleared by the liver, the carcinoid syndrome is a late manifestation of these tumors, appearing only after hepatic metastases have occurred. Exceptions are carcinoid tumors arising in the bronchial tree or the gonads, areas that drain into the systemic circulation, so patients may have carcinoid syndrome before tumor metastasis.

Production and metabolism of serotonin differ relative to the tissue of origin of the tumor. Tumors of mid-gut origin contain and release large quantities of 5-HT; this may not be fully reflected in the amount of the metabolite 5-HIAA in urine because little 5-HT is metabolized. Tumors from fore-gut cells also produce large amounts of 5-HT which is oxidized within the tumor to 5-HIAA. With these fore-gut tumors, urinary excretion of 5-HIAA is often much higher than would be expected from the clinical presentation. Tumors from hind-gut cells only rarely produce excess 5-HT or 5-HIAA.

Clinical Presentation

Patients with carcinoid tumors arising in the small intestine, appendix, or rectum usually present with local manifestations of the tumor including bleeding, obstruction, or metastases, without humoral manifestations.

The classic clinical presentation of carcinoid syndrome includes pronounced flushing, bronchial constriction, diarrhea, and cardiac valvular lesions, often associated with right-sided heart failure. Severe hypotension may occur. Serotonin excess accounts for the diarrhea associated with this tumor, but other substances are involved in the other clinical manifestations. Carcinoid tumors often produce excesses of substances such as histamine, catecholamines, prostaglandins, vasoactive peptides, kallikrein, substance P, neurotensin, ACTH, growth hormone, and insulin. Carcinoid tumors may also be associated with multiple endocrine neoplasia.

Diagnosis of Carcinoid Tumors

Patients with functioning carcinoid tumors usually have striking increases in urinary excretion of 5-HIAA (>25 mg/d; normal is <9 mg/d). If a borderline elevation of 5-HIAA is found (6 to 25 mg/d), repeat collections should be made and care taken to avoid the patient's use of food and medications that might elevate 5-HIAA (e.g., pineapples, avocados, bananas, walnuts, chocolate, guaifenesin, and reserpine). Nontropical sprue may cause a slight increase in urinary 5-HIAA. 5-HIAA levels are lowered by phenothiazines, in renal insufficiency, and after small bowel resection.

When 5-HIAA in urine is normal, as may be the case with mid-gut carcinoid tumors when serotonin is produced in excess but not metabolized, assay for blood or urine levels of 5-hydroxytryptophan (5-HTP) or 5-HT is sometimes needed to document the diagnosis of carcinoid syndrome. Measurement of other compounds such as substance P and neurotensin do not add to the diagnostic evaluation for carcinoid tumors.

If carcinoid syndrome is present and serotonin or 5-HIAA excess has been shown, there are three possibilities: (1) tumor metastasis to the liver, in which case CT scan will at least show the metastases and perhaps the primary tumor as well; (2) carcinoid of the gonads; or (3) bronchial carcinoid. Demonstration of tumors in these latter sites may be difficult, with CT or other imaging techniques as well as direct visualization by bronchoscopy or laparoscopy being useful.

Treatment of Carcinoid Tumors

Surgical resection of the primary carcinoid tumor is the treatment of choice. Many carcinoid tumors are malignant and metastasize early, in which case surgical cure is not possible. However, the course of malignant carcinoid is often slow, with palliation giving effective tumor control for months or years.

Hepatic metastases may be reduced in bulk by procedures that interfere with their arterial blood supply such as ligation or radiographically controlled embolization. Chemotherapeutic agents such as streptozotocin, 5-fluorouracil, cytoxan, and doxorubicin have produced some responses. The best chemotherapeutic agent appears to be a long acting somatostatin analogue, a drug with minimal toxicity which relieves many or all of the symptoms of carcinoid syndrome and produces substantial tumor shrinkage.

Carcinoid flushing can usually be managed with histamine (H1 or H2) blocking agents. Cyproheptadine, a drug with both antihistamine and antiserotonin properties may be useful for flushing and diarrhea.

Feldman JM, O'Dorisio TM: Role of neuropeptides and serotonin in the diagnosis of carcinoid tumors. Am J Med 1986; *81*(suppl 6B):41–48.

Kvols LK: Metastatic carcinoid tumors and the carcinoid syndrome: A selective review of chemotherapy and hormonal therapy. Am J Med 1986; *81*(suppl 6B):49–55.

Kvols LK, Moertel CG, O'Connell MJ, et al.: Treatment of malignant carcinoid syndrome: Evaluation of a long-acting somatostatin analogue. N Engl J Med 1986; *315*:663–666.

Oates JA: The carcinoid syndrome. N Engl J Med 1986; *315*:702–704.

GASTROINTESTINAL HORMONES

A wide variety of hormones are produced throughout the gastrointestinal tract. These hormones are involved in various aspects of the digestive process. The main clinical significance of these hormones is their production by neoplasms. Those hormone-secreting neoplasms that arise in the pancreas are shown in Table 11–3. The most frequent of these uncommon neoplasms are tumors secreting gastrin, VIP, and pancreatic polypeptide. The diagnosis and treatment of these rare tumors are covered in recent review articles and symposia.

Friesen SR: Tumors of the endocrine pancreas. N Engl J Med 1982; *306*:580–590.
Jensen RT (moderator): Zollinger-Ellison syndrome: Current concepts and management. Ann Intern Med 1983; *98*:59–75.
O'Dorisio TM: Gut endocrinology: Clinical and therapeutic impact. Am J Med 1986; *81*:(suppl 6B):1–7.
Romanus ME, Neal JA, Dilley WG, et al.: Comparison of four provocative tests for the diagnosis of gastrinoma. Ann Surg 1983; *197*:608–617.
Gastrointestinal endocrine tumors: Diagnosis and management. Am J Med 1987; *82*:(suppl 5B):1–99.

AUTOIMMUNITY IN ENDOCRINOLOGY

Autoimmunity is involved in the pathogenesis of many endocrine diseases, both commonly occurring ones like type I diabetes mellitus, Graves' hyperthyroidism, and Hashimoto's thyroiditis, and uncommon ones as well. A patient with one autoimmune endocrine disorder is at increased risk for a second or even a third. The triad of type I diabetes mellitus, Hashimoto's thyroiditis, and Addison's disease is known as Schmidt's syndrome. Patients with autoimmune endocrine diseases are also at increased risk for a variety of nonendocrine autoimmune diseases. Table 11–4 shows these autoimmune disorders.

The general mechanism of these disorders appears to be a deficit in immune surveillance, related in part to specific HLA types that enhance antigen presentation and overwhelm suppressor T cells. The resulting autoantibodies may bind and activate hormone receptors (e.g., antibodies in Graves' disease activate the TSH receptor on thyroid cells) or attract killer cells to destroy endocrine tissue (e.g., Hashimoto's thyroiditis, type I diabetes mellitus). Antibodies have also been identified that bind with receptors and block hormone binding (atrophic

Table 11–3.   Clinical Features of Non-Insulin-Producing Islet Cell Tumors

Tumor Syndrome	Clinical Features	Diagnostic Features*
Glucagonoma	Necrolytic migratory erythema, mild diabetes, psychiatric disturbances, diarrhea, venous thrombosis	Excessive glucagon release after intravenous administration of tolbutamide
Somatostatinoma	Dyspepsia, diabetes, gallstones, steatorrhea, hypochlorhydria	Hyperglycemia without ketonemia; stool weight usually 400 to 800 g per day, stool fat 10 to 30 g per day
PPoma	None recognized (secretory diarrhea in one case)	None known for pure PPoma
Gastrinoma	Severe peptic ulcer disease, secretory diarrhea	Serum gastrin increase after intravenous administration of secretin; high basal and peak acid secretion; secretory diarrhea stops with histamine (H_2)-receptor antagonist therapy
VIPoma	Large-volume secretory diarrhea, hypokalemia, metabolic acidosis, hypochlorhydria	Stool electrolytes (sodium plus potassium times two) account for osmolality of stool water without gap; fecal pH as high as 8.0 on fasting (colonic bicarbonate secretion); concomitant elevation of plasma PHM (peptide histidine methionine)
Calcitoninoma	Diarrhea	Secretory diarrhea while fasting; additional osmotic component while eating (decreased small-bowel transit time)
Neurotensinoma	Esophageal reflux (in one case)	None known for pure neurotensinoma
Pancreatic GRFoma	Acromegaly	Normal sella; normal findings on computerized tomographic scan of head; no growth hormone release by exogenous GRF (pituitary tumors respond)

*Other than elevated basal plasma peptide concentration.
(Used by permission from Krejs GJ: Gastrointestinal endocrine tumors. Am J Med 1987: *82*(suppl 5B):1–3.)

Table 11–4. Autoimmune Diseases

Endocrine	*Nonendocrine*
Type I diabetes mellitus	Pernicious anemia
Graves' disease	Vitiligo
Hashimoto's thyroiditis	Myasthenia gravis
Addison's disease	Chronic active hepatitis
Autoimmune ovarian failure	Rheumatoid arthritis
Autoimmune parathyroid failure	
Autoimmune pituitary failure	

goiter), or bind with receptors and activate one function but not others (thyroid growth-stimulating immunoglobulins).

There are studies underway to see if the course of autoimmune glandular destruction can be aborted with immunosuppressive agents. At present, treatment of autoimmune endocrine diseases is limited to replacement of deficient hormones or, in the case of endocrine hyperfunction, glandular ablation or medical inhibition of hormone synthesis or action.

Konishi J, Iida Y, Kasagi K et al.: Primary myxedema with thyrotrophin-binding inhibitor immunoglobulins: Clinical and laboratory findings in 15 patients. Ann Intern Med 1985; *103*:26–31.

Nichols WS, Nakamura RM: Antibody patterns in autoimmune disease. Lab Management 1984; *22*:39–45.

Strakosch SR, Wenzel BE, Row VV, et al.: Immunology of autoimmune thyroid diseases. N Engl J Med 1982; *307*:1499–1507.

Trence DL, Morley JE, Handwerger BS: Polyglandular autoimmune syndromes. Am J Med 1984; *77*:107–116.

Volpe R: Immunoregulation in autoimmune thyroid disease. N Engl J Med 1987; *316*:44–46.

12

Testing Protocols

ACTH (COSYNTROPIN) TEST FOR ADRENAL RESERVE

Rationale. In normal subjects, cosyntropin (a short-acting but potent form of ACTH) causes a rapid rise in serum cortisol. Patients with primary adrenal insufficiency show no change in serum cortisol after ACTH. Patients with secondary adrenal insufficiency may show a slight rise in serum cortisol but not of normal magnitude. Be certain not to use depot forms of ACTH or ACTH of bovine origin for this test.

Procedure. A baseline sample is drawn for serum cortisol. 250 μg of cosyntropin (1–24 ACTH) is given IM or IV. Further samples for serum cortisol are drawn 30 and/or 60 min after injection.

Interpretation. In normals, serum serum cortisol rises >7 μg/dL, peak serum cortisol is >20 mg/dL. The rise may be less if the basal serum cortisol is high due to stress.

Hjortrup A, Kehlet H, Lindholm J, et al.: Value of the 30-minute adrenocorticotropin (ACTH) test in demonstrating hypothalamic-pituitary-adrenocortical insufficiency after acute ACTH deprivation. J Clin Endocrinol Metab 1983; 57:668–670.
May ME, Carey RM: Rapid adrenocorticotropic hormone test in practice: retrospective review. Am J Med 1985; 79:679–684.

CALCIUM/PENTAGASTRIN STIMULATION FOR CALCITONIN (MEDULLARY CARCINOMA OF THE THYROID)

Rationale. In patients with early medullary carcinoma of the thyroid (or hyperplasia of calcitonin-producing cells, a premalignant lesion), basal levels of calcitonin may be normal. In these patients, stimulation with calcium, pentagastrin, or both will show an exaggerated response. Some authorities prefer to use a calcium challenge, others use pentagastrin, and some use both. This testing approach is primarily useful for surveillance of relatives in families with multiple endocrine neoplasia syndromes IIa and IIb.

Procedure. A basal blood sample is obtained for calcitonin measurement. Calcium 2 mg/kg body weight is given intravenously over 50 seconds (10 mL 10% calcium gluconate contains 95 mg calcium). For the combined test, pentagastrin 0.5 µg/kg bodyweight is given IV over 10 sec. Samples for calcitonin are drawn at 1, 2.5, 4, and 6 min.

Interpretation. Calcitonin levels should remain within the normal range or rise only slightly in normals. Peak values over 1 ng/mL are indicative of C-cell malignancy.

Hennessey JF, Wells SA Jr, Ontjes DA, et al.: A comparison of pentagastrin injection and calcium infusion as provocative agents for the detection of medullary carcinoma of the thyroid. J Clin Endocrinol Metab 1974; *39*:487–495.

Rude RK, Singer FR: Comparison of serum calcitonin levels after a 1-minute calcium injection and after pentagastrin injection in the diagnosis of medullary thyroid carcinoma. J Clin Endocrinol Metab 1977; *44*:980–983.

CLONIDINE SUPPRESSION TEST FOR PHEOCHROMOCYTOMA

Rationale. Clonidine, a centrally acting alpha adrenergic antagonist, inhibits norepinephrine release in normal subjects but not in patients with pheochromocytoma.

Procedure. The test is best done in the morning after an overnight fast. The patient remains recumbent through the entire procedure. Blood is drawn for plasma catecholamine determination 30 min after insertion of an indwelling needle for repeated sampling. Clonidine, 0.3 mg, is given orally and a repeat sample for plasma catecholamines drawn 3 h later.

Interpretation. Plasma norepinephrine should be within the established normal range at 3 h. Plasma norepinephrine above normal at 3 h is highly suggestive of pheochromocytoma.

Bravo EL, Tarazi RC, Fouad FM, et al.: Clonidine-suppression test: A useful aid in the diagnosis of pheochromocytoma. N Engl J Med 1981; *305*:623–626.

DEXAMETHASONE SUPPRESSION TEST (HIGH DOSE) FOR CUSHING'S SYNDROME

Rationale. Patients with Cushing's disease (due to an ACTH-producing pituitary adenoma) usually show suppression of cortisol with high-dose dexamethasone. Patients with Cushing's syndrome due to other causes (adrenal adenoma or carcinoma, ectopic production of ACTH) usually do not have a significant change in cortisol under these conditions.

Procedure. Twenty-four-hour urine collections are obtained daily for 4 d for free cortisol and 17-hydroxysteroid determinations. Dexamethasone, 2.0 mg orally every 6 h, is begun at 0800 h on day 3 and continued for 8 doses. Free cortisol, 17-hydroxysteroids, and creatinine are measured in each 24-h sample. Other measurements include serum cortisol at 0800 h and 2000 h on day 1 or 2 to look for diurnal variation, and at 0800 h on day 5 to look for suppression.

Interpretation. Patients with Cushing's disease due to an ACTH-secreting pituitary adenoma will usually show (1) suppression of urine free cortisol and 17-hydroxysteroid excretion >50% of baseline by day 4, (2) lack of diurnal variation in serum cortisol, and (3) serum cortisol <10 μg/dL at 0800 h on day 5.

Liddle GW: Tests of pituitary-adrenal suppressibility in the diagnosis of Cushing's syndrome, J Clin Endocrinol Metab 1960; *20*:1539–1560.

DEXAMETHASONE SUPPRESSION TEST (LOW DOSE) FOR CUSHING'S SYNDROME

Rationale. Normal subjects show lowering of serum and urinary cortisol and metabolites under the conditions of low-dose dexamethasone suppression. Patients with Cushing's syndrome usually show persistent elevation of cortisol under these conditions.

Procedure. Twenty-four-hour urine samples are collected daily for 4 consecutive days. Dexamethasone 0.5 mg given orally every 6 h is begun at 0800 h on day 3 and continued for 8 doses. Free cortisol, 17-hydroxysteroids, and creatinine are measured in each 24-h urine sample. Other measurements include serum cortisol at 0800 h and 2000 h on day 1 or 2 to look for diurnal variation and serum cortisol at 0800 h on day 5 to look for suppression.

Interpretation. Urine free cortisol should be <50% of the upper limit of normal on day 4 and urine 17-hydroxysteroids

<4 mg/g of creatinine. Serum cortisol on day 4 should be <5 µg/dL. With normal diurnal variation, serum cortisol at 2000 h should be two-thirds the value at 0800 h. Patients with Cushing's syndrome will usually not show diurnal rhythm or suppression of serum or urine steroids with low-dose dexamethasone. Patients taking diphenylhydantoin or phenobarbital, or both, metabolize dexamethasone more rapidly than normal and may not show suppression.

Liddle GW: Tests of pituitary-adrenal suppressibility in the diagnosis of Cushing's syndrome, J Clin Endocrinol Metab 1960; *20*:1539–1560.

DEXAMETHASONE SUPPRESSION TEST (OVERNIGHT) FOR CUSHING'S SYNDROME

Rationale. Dexamethasone, a potent cortisol analog, suppresses cortisol production in normal subjects but not in patients with Cushing's syndrome.

Procedure. Dexamethasone 1.0 mg is given orallly at 2300 h, along with a sedative (such as flurazepam [Dalmane] 15 or 30 mg). Blood is drawn for determination of serum cortisol at 0700 h.

Interpretation. Normally, serum cortisol will be ≤5 µg/dL the morning after 1 mg of dexamethasone. Serum cortisol >10 µg/dL is seen in Cushing's syndrome, but may also be seen due to stress, failure to take the dexamethasone, treatment with diphenylhydantoin or phenobarbital (enhancement of dexamethasone metabolism), or endogenous depression.

Pavlatos FC, Smilo RP, Forsham PF: A rapid screening test for Cushing's syndrome. JAMA 1965; *193*:96–99.

FLUDROCORTISONE SUPPRESSION TEST FOR HYPERALDOSTERONISM

Rationale. Fludrocortisone, a potent mineralocorticoid, will suppress aldosterone production in normal subjects but not in subjects with primary aldosteronism.

Procedure. Hypokalemia must be corrected before starting this test, and serum potassium monitored during the test. Fludrocortisone, 0.1 mg every 6 h, is given orally for 3 d; 24-h urine collections for aldosterone are obtained.

Interpretation. Normal subjects have urine aldosterone ≤20 μg on day 3. Patients with primary aldosteronism have urine aldosterone >20 μg/d.

Biglieri EG, Stockigt Jr, Schambelan M: A preliminary evaluation for primary aldosteronism. Arch Intern Med 1970; *126*:1004–1007.

FUROSEMIDE STIMULATION TEST FOR PLASMA RENIN ACTIVITY

Rationale. Plasma renin activity varies with hydration and sodium intake. Furosemide, a potent diuretic, provides a stimulus to increase plasma renin activity.

Procedure. Furosemide 60 mg is given orally at 0700 h. The subject remains upright (seated or standing) until blood is drawn at 1200 h for determination of plasma renin activity.

Interpretation. Responses must be defined for the assay technique employed. Patients with renovascular hypertension show values approximately five times normal. Patients with primary aldosteronism usually have plasma renin activity below the level of assay sensitivity. Figure 7–6 shows typical responses.

Wallach L, Nyari I, Dawson KG: Stimulated renin: A screening test for hypertension. Ann Intern Med 1975; *82*:27–34.

GESTATIONAL DIABETES SCREENING TEST

Rationale. All pregnant women should be screened for gestational diabetes in the first trimester. Screening can be done at any time of the day, without regard for previous meals, by measuring serum glucose after an oral glucose load. Women with a positive screening test should have an oral glucose tolerance test (protocol p. 212). Since glucose tolerance deteriorates during the last trimester of pregnancy, high-risk women with a normal screen or GTT in the first trimester should be retested at about 32 weeks gestation.

Procedure. A 50-g glucose load is given orally and serum glucose determined 1 h later.

Interpretation. Serum glucose >140 mg/dL is positive.

American Diabetes Association: Gestational diabetes mellitus. Ann Intern Med 1986; *105*:461.

GLUCOSE SUPPRESSION OF GROWTH HORMONE

Rationale. In normal subjects but not in patients with acromegaly, growth hormone is suppressed after oral administration of glucose.

Procedure. Begin after an overnight fast. Ideally, the patient should be kept at bed rest, since GH increases after exercise. However, this test usually gives appropriate results in ambulatory subjects. After collecting a baseline sample for GH measurement, 100 g glucose solution is given orally; GH is measured again on a sample collected 60 min later. The baseline GH measurement is not essential.

Interpretation. GH should fall to <5 ng/mL (typically <1 ng/mL); subjects with acromegaly fail to show any decrease in GH and may show a paradoxical rise.

Earll JM, Sparks LL, Forsham PH: Glucose suppression of serum growth hormone in the diagnosis of acromegaly. JAMA 1967; *201*:134–136.

GLUCOSE TOLERANCE TEST FOR GESTATIONAL DIABETES MELLITUS

Rationale. Detection and effective treatment of gestational diabetes substantially reduces or eliminates risks to the fetus. Patients with a positive screening test (protocol p. 211) should have an oral glucose tolerance test. For 3 d before the test, a diet containing at least 150 g of carbohydrate daily should be ingested.

Procedure. After drawing a sample for fasting serum glucose, 100 g of an oral glucose solution is given and samples for serum glucose drawn hourly for 3 hours.

Interpretation. The results are interpreted using the criteria of O'Sullivan and Mahan, 1964 (Table 9–5, p. 168).

National Diabetes Data Group: Classification and diagnosis of diabetes mellitus and other categories of glucose intolerance. Diabetes. 1979; *28*:1039–1057.

O'Sullivan JB, Mahan C: Criteria for oral glucose tolerance test in pregnancy. Diabetes 1964; *13*:278–285.

GLUCOSE TOLERANCE TEST FOR NONINSULIN-DEPENDENT DIABETES MELLITUS

Rationale. NIDDM can be diagnosed prior to the development of fasting hyperglycemia by demonstrating glucose intolerance. Since there is no specific treatment for the earliest stages of

NIDDM, OGTT diagnosis is usually unnecessary. Many factors can impair glucose tolerance temporarily (Table 9–4), p. 167). If an OGTT is to be done, as many of these factors as possible should be eliminated.

Procedure. Only healthy, ambulatory subjects should be tested. At least 3 d of unrestricted diet and activity should precede the test, with the diet containing at least 150 g of carbohydrate a day. Medications known to impair glucose tolerance (e.g., diuretics, estrogens, steroids) should be stopped. After drawing a fasting sample for serum glucose, an oral glucose load of 75 g is given. Additional samples are drawn at 1 and 2 h.

Interpretation. Criteria for the diagnosis of NIDDM are shown in Table 9–3, p. 166.

National Diabetes Data Group: Classification and diagnosis of diabetes mellitus and other categories of glucose intolerance. Diabetes 1979; *28*:1039–1057.

GONADOTROPIN-RELEASING HORMONE (GnRH) STIMULATION FOR LH AND FSH RESERVE

Rationale. The hypothalamic releasing hormone, GnRH, stimulates release of both LH and FSH in normal individuals. Subnormal responses are seen in some patients with pituitary or hypothalamic disorders. However, the magnitude of LH and FSH response to GnRH is usually predictable from the basal LH and FSH levels. This test may be useful in patients where the clinical picture and basal gonadotropin measurements are inconclusive or confusing.

Procedure. The test may be performed without regard for previous feeding or time of day. After baseline samples are obtained for LH and/or FSH determination, 100 μg GnRH is given IV. Samples for LH and/or FSH should be drawn every 15 to 30 min for 1 to 2 h.

Interpretation. LH should increase by 3- to 10-fold. The FSH response is of lesser magnitude, usually a 1.5- to 3-fold increase. The peak responses for both LH and FSH occur between 15 and 30 min. Patients with primary hypogonadism show an exaggerated response. Patients with pituitary disorders may have normal, diminished, or absent responses. In patients with hypothalamic disorders, the response may be exaggerated, normal, diminished, or absent.

Mortimer RH, Besser GM, McNeilly AS, et al.: Luteinizing hormone and follicle stimulating hormone releasing hormone test in patients with hypothalamic-pituitary-gonadal dysfunction. Br Med J 1973; *4*:73–75.

Orry SJ: Clinical uses of luteinizing hormone-releasing hormone. Fertil Steril 1983; *39*:577–591.

GONADOTROPIN STIMULATION (hCG) FOR TESTOSTERONE RESERVE

Rationale. In prepubertal boys, administration of chorionic gonadotropin (hCG) should stimulate production of testosterone and increase testicular size. This is useful in evaluation of males with no palpable gonadal tissue in the scrotal sac.

Procedure. Blood is drawn for testosterone measurement; hCG 5000 U is given intramuscularly (day 0) and a second sample for testosterone drawn 4 d later.

Interpretation. Serum testosterone should rise into the normal adult range (usually 300 to 1000 ng/dL) on day 4. No response indicates absence of functioning testicular tissue. Subnormal responses may be seen in hypogonadotropic hypogonadism. If cryptorchidism is being considered, physical examination or ultrasound may reveal testicular tissue on day 4.

Dunkel L, Perheentupa J, Sorva R: Single versus repeated dose human chorionic gonadotropin stimulation in the differential diagnosis of hypogonadotropic hypogonadism. J Clin Endocrinol Metab 1985; *60*:333–337.

Grant DB, Laurance BM, Atherden SM, et al.: hCG Stimulation test in children with abnormal sexual development. Arch Dis Child 1976; *51*:596–602.

INSULIN TOLERANCE TEST FOR GH AND/OR ACTH RESERVE

Rationale. Stress triggers the release of many hormones, among them growth hormone and ACTH. In this test, the stress is hypoglycemia induced by insulin. GH is measured directly and cortisol is used as the indicator of ACTH response. This test may be combined with the hypothalamic releasing factors TRH and GnRH for a "cocktail" test of all anterior pituitary hormones.

Procedure. Begin after an overnight fast with the patient at bed rest. An indwelling needle or IV line must be inserted for delivery of medication and for administration of dextrose when hypoglycemia occurs. Sampling is begun after a 30-min rest period. Baseline samples are drawn for determination of glucose, growth hormone, and cortisol (and other hormones if other releasing factors are given). Regular insulin, 0.1 to 0.15 U/kg body weight, is given intravenously. Samples are obtained at 30, 60, and 90 min for glucose, growth hormone, and cortisol. To be certain an adequate stress has occurred, the patient must become symptomatic (sweating, tremor) or the glucose concentration must fall to <40 mg/dL; additional intravenous insulin may be given if this has not occurred by 30 min. The physician should stay in attendance throughout the test; 50% dextrose for intravenous administration must be kept on hand and given when the patient becomes symptomatic from hypoglycemia. Once the stress has occurred, hypoglycemia may be reversed without interfering with the results.

Interpretation. Assuming an adequate stress has been achieved, cortisol should increase by >7 μg/dL to a peak value >20 μg/dL. Growth hormone should rise to >7 ng/mL. Failure to respond may be due to pituitary hormone deficiency or a hypothalamic lesion.

Eddy RL, Gilliland PF, Ibarra JD, et al.: Human growth hormone release: comparison of provocative test procedures. Am J Med 1974; *56*:179–185.

Landon J, Wynn V, James VHT: The adrenocortical response to insulin-induced hypoglycemia. J Endocrinol 1963; *27*:183–192.

L-DOPA SCREENING FOR GROWTH HORMONE RESERVE

Rationale. L-Dopa stimulates a rise in GH in normal individuals but not in patients with GH deficiency.

Procedure. L-Dopa, 250 mg tid, is given orally with meals for 2 d as a "priming" preparation. The stimulus dose of L-dopa, 500 mg/1.73 m², is given with lunch and a sample drawn for GH measurement 60 min later.

Interpretation. GH should rise to over 10 ng/mL in normals. A normal response excludes GH deficiency. However, a subnormal response may be seen in up to 20% of normal individuals, so a subnormal response must be confirmed with additional testing (insulin tolerance test, 24-h GH profile, etc.)

Eddy RL, Gilliland PF, Ibarra JD, et al.: Human growth hormone release: comparison of provocative test procedures. Am J Med 1974; *56*:179–185.

MEAL TOLERANCE TEST FOR "REACTIVE HYPOGLYCEMIA"

Rationale. Several hours after a meal, patients with "reactive" or alimentary hypoglycemia will show a fall in serum glucose and adrenergic symptoms of hypoglycemia. An oral glucose load is an artificial situation and may produce a fall in serum glucose in healthy individuals, so the glucose tolerance test should be avoided.

Procedure. Pre-test conditions for the oral glucose tolerance test should be met (Table 9–4, p. 167). After a fasting blood sample is obtained, the patient eats a standard meal: 6 oz of unsweetened orange juice, 8 oz of cornflakes or oatmeal, 8 oz of low fat milk, 1 tbsp of sugar, 2 slices of toast, tea or decaffeinated coffee ad lib. Additional samples for serum glucose are drawn every 30 min for 5 h.

Interpretation. There are no fixed criteria for the diagnosis of alimentary hypoglycemia. This diagnosis is likely if serum glucose drops below 60 mg/dL and the patient has adrenergic symptoms of hypoglycemia (Table 9–10, p. 182).

Charles MA, Hofeldt F, Shackelford A, et al.: Comparison of oral glucose tolerance tests and mixed meals in patients with apparent postabsorptive hypoglycemia: absence of hypoglycemia after meals. Diabetes 1981; *30*:465–470.

Hogan MJ, Service FJ, Sharborough FW, et al.: Oral glucose tolerance test compared with a mixed meal in the diagnosis of reactive hypoglycemia: A caveat on stimulation. Mayo Clin Proc 1983; *58*:491–496.

METYRAPONE TEST (OVERNIGHT) FOR ACTH RESERVE

Rationale. Metyrapone inhibits 11-hydroxylase activity, the enzyme step immediately preceding cortisol synthesis. As the level of cortisol falls, negative feedback on the pituitary is diminished, causing release of ACTH. ACTH acts on the adrenal cortex, producing a rise in 11-deoxycortisol, the compound immediately preceding cortisol in the biosynthetic pathway.

Procedure. Metyrapone (3 g) is given orally at 2300 h with milk or a snack to delay absorption. Blood is drawn at 0700 h the next day for determination of 11-deoxycortisol and cortisol.

Interpretation. 11-Deoxycortisol normally rises to >7 μg/dL after metyrapone. Failure to respond may be seen in pituitary or hypothalamic disease or with inadequate enzyme blockade (serum cortisol >3 μg/dL). (11-Deoxycortisol <7 μg/dL and simultaneous serum cortisol >3 µg/dl indicate inadequate block-ade.)

Spark RF: Simplified assessment of pituitary-adrenal reserve: measurement of serum 11-deoxycortisol and cortisol after metyrapone. Ann Intern Med 1971; *75*:717–720.

RENAL VEIN RENINS FOR RENAL ARTERY STENOSIS

Rationale. In renovascular hypertension plasma renin activity is higher in the renal vein on the involved side.

Procedure. The patient should be on a low-sodium, high-potassium diet and a diuretic for 3 d before the procedure. Under fluoroscopic guidance, percutaneous catheterization is performed and samples obtained from both renal veins and inferior vena cava for plasma renin activity.

Interpretation. Various criteria have been suggested for interpretation. A ratio of plasma renin activity >1.5 comparing the affected to unaffected side suggests functionally significant renovascular disease. More specific criteria may be found in the report of the Working Group.

Working Group on Renovascular Hypertension: Detection, evaluation, and treatment of renovascular hypertension: Final report. Arch Intern Med 1987; *147*:820–829.

SALINE INFUSION TEST FOR DIABETES INSIPIDUS

Rationale. Increased plasma osmolality is a strong stimulus for release of ADH. Administration of hypertonic saline solution intravenously to produce a hyperosmolar state causes a rise in plasma ADH that can be plotted against plasma osmolality and compared with a nomogram (Fig. 3–1).

Procedure. Intravenous 3% saline is begun at a minimum rate to maintain flow. Baseline samples are drawn for plasma osmolality and ADH at -15 m and 0 time. The rate of 3% saline is maintained for 2 h with an infusion pump at 0.1 mL/kg/min and samples drawn for plasma osmolality and ADH every 15 min.

Interpretation. In normal subjects plasma ADH will be >7 pg/mL when plasma osmolality is ≥310 mOsm/L. Figure 3–1 shows typical responses for patients with disorders of ADH secretion or action.

Zerbe RL, Robertson GL: A comparison of plasma vasopressin measurements with a standard indirect test in the differential diagnosis of polyuria. N Engl J Med 1981; *305*:1539–1546.

SALINE SUPPRESSION TEST FOR HYPERALDOSTERONISM

Rationale. Rapid volume expansion with intravenous saline should suppress plasma aldosterone in normal subjects but not in patients with primary aldosteronism.

Procedure. Care must be taken to ensure that the subject is not hypokalemic before starting the test. Begin test in the morning, before breakfast, after the patient has been upright for 2 h. Blood is drawn for determination of plasma aldosterone. The subject then assumes a supine position and 2 L of 0.9% saline is infused over 4 h. Blood is drawn for plasma aldosterone at the end of the infusion.

Interpretation. Normal individuals show plasma aldosterone ≤5 ng/dL after saline infusion. Levels >5 ng/dL are usually seen in patients with primary aldosteronism.

Kem DC, Weinberger MH, Mayes DM, et al.: Saline suppression of plasma aldosterone in hypertension. Arch Intern Med 1971; *128*:380–386.

TRH STIMULATION OF TSH RELEASE

Rationale. The pituitary is exquisitely sensitive to changes in thyroid hormones. When thyroid hormones rise above normal, TSH release is reduced or blocked; when thyroid hormones fall below normal, TSH release in response to TRH is exaggerated.

Procedure. No patient preparation is necessary. A baseline sample is collected for TSH determination (and T_4, if not already done); 500 μg TRH is given IV and repeat samples drawn for TSH 30 and 60 min after injection.

Interpretation. A normal response is a 5- to 10-fold rise of TSH, with the peak value at 30 min. Blunted or flat responses are seen in hyperthyroidism (usually with high T_4 and T_3), or in hypothyroidism secondary to hypopituitarism (usually with a low T_4). An exaggerated rise (peak TSH >35 mU/mL is seen in early primary hypothyroidism. Patients with hypothyroidism secondary to hypothalmic disorders may show a response of normal magnitude but a delayed peak.

Hershman JM: Clinical application of thyrotropin-releasing hormone. N Engl J Med 1974; *290*:886–889.
Jackson IMD: Thyrotropin-releasing hormone. N Engl J Med 1982; *306*:145–154.

WATER DEPRIVATION TEST FOR DIABETES INSIPIDUS AND OTHER POLYURIC DISORDERS

Rationale. Dehydration is a strong stimulus for ADH release which can be assessed indirectly by measuring urine osmolality or directly by measuring plasma ADH. If urine remains hypoosmolar during water deprivation, diabetes insipidus is present. Once urine osmolality has stabilized during dehydration, administration of ADH helps differentiate central diabetes insipidus from nephrogenic diabetes insipidus.

Procedure. The patient is weighed at 2200 h, at which time plasma and urine samples are collected for sodium concentration and osmolality. No oral intake is allowed until the test is terminated. Care is taken to be sure the patient's body weight does not fall by ≥5% during the test. Beginning at 0600 h the patient is again weighed and hourly urine collections begun for measurement of volume and determination of osmolality. When urine osmolality is stable (a change of ≤30 mOsm/L for two consecutive hours, which usually takes 8 to 12 h), samples are collected for plasma osmolality (and plasma ADH, if desired). Aqueous vasopressin, 5 units, is given subcutaneously and urine osmolality measured 1 h later.

Interpretation. Normal individuals will lose ≤3% of body weight, will maintain a normal plasma sodium osmolality, and will produce a concentrated urine (osmolality ≥400 mOsm/L), with no further increase in urine osmolality after ADH administration. Patients with *central diabetes insipidus* show an increase in plasma osmolality and serum sodium; their urine will be less concentrated than normal (≤400 mOsm/L; often less than plasma), and urine osmolality increases ≥10% after ADH administration. Patients with *nephrogenic diabetes insipidus* show plasma and urine osmolalities similar to patients with central DI but no increase in urine osmolality after ADH injection. In *psychogenic polydipsia,* because of reduced concentrations of solutes in the renal medulla, a subnormal response may be seen unless the period of water deprivation is prolonged.

Miller M, Dalakos T, Moses AM, et al.: Recognition of partial defects in antidiuretic hormone secretion. Ann Intern Med 1970; *73*:721–729.

Price JDE, Lauener RW: Serum and urine osmolalities in the differential diagnosis of polyuric states. J Clin Endocrinol Metab 1966; *26*:143–148.

WATER LOADING TEST FOR SIADH

Rationale. An excess of antidiuretic hormone leads to hyponatremia by interfering with the ability of the kidneys to excrete a water load normally. This test is useful if SIADH is suspected in a patient with normal or near normal serum sodium and osmolality, or in patients with "reset osmostat." This test should not be done in patients who are already significantly hyponatremic because of the danger that the water load will worsen the hyponatremia.

Procedure. Begin in the morning 2 h after a light breakfast. Plasma and urine osmolality are measured. The patient is given water to drink over a 15- to 30-min period, 20 mL/kg; lightly salted crackers may be given with the water if needed. The patient is kept recumbent, with samples taken hourly for the next 4 h for plasma and urine osmolality. Total urine output is measured.

Interpretation. Plasma osmolality should decrease by ≥ 5 mOsm/L and urine osmolality should drop to ≤ 100 mOsm/L, with $\geq 90\%$ of the water load excreted in 4 h. SIADH is characterized by $<90\%$ of the water load being excreted and urine osmolality remaining >100 mOsm/L. Plasma ADH may be measured 90 or 120 min after the water load as additional confirmation of the diagnosis. Subnormal responses are seen with glucocorticoid deficiency, hypothyroidism, and renal diseases.

Moses AM, Gabrilove JL, Soffer LJ: Simplified water loading test in hypoadrenocorticism and hypothyroidism. J Clin Endocrinol Metab 1955; *18*:1413–1417.

Robertson GL: Posterior pituitary. *In* Felig P, Baxter JD, Broadus AE, Frohman LA (eds): Endocrinology and Metabolism, 2nd ed. New York, McGraw-Hill, 1987, p 375.

INDEX

Numerals in *italics* indicate a figure; "t" following a page number indicates a table.